PROMOTING PARTNERSHIP FOR HEALTH

Interprofessional Teamwork for Health and Social Care

PROMOTING PARTNERSHIP
FOR HEALTH

Interprofessional Teamwork for Health and Social Care

Scott Reeves

Simon Lewin

Sherry Espin

Merrick Zwarenstein

Series Editor: Hugh Barr

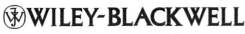

WILEY-BLACKWELL

A John Wiley & Sons, Ltd., Publication

CAIPE

Registered office
John Wiley & Sons Ltd, The Atrium, Southern Gate, Chichester, West Sussex, PO19 8SQ, United Kingdom

Editorial offices
9600 Garsington Road, Oxford, OX4 2DQ, United Kingdom
2121 State Avenue, Ames, Iowa 50014-8300, USA

For details of our global editorial offices, for customer services and for information about how to apply for permission to reuse the copyright material in this book please see our website at www.wiley.com/wiley-blackwell.

Library of Congress Cataloging-in-Publication Data

Interprofessional teamwork for health and social care / Scott Reeves ... [et al.].
    p. ; cm. – (Promoting partnership for health)
  Includes bibliographical references and index.
  ISBN 978-1-4051-8191-4 (hardback : alk. paper)   1. Health care teams.
I. Reeves, Scott, 1967–   II. Series: Promoting partnership for health.
  [DNLM: 1. Patient Care Team.   2. Delivery of Health Care–organization & administration.   3. Interprofessional Relations.   4. Social Work–methods.
W 84.8 I613 2010]
  R729.5.H4I583 2010
  362.1–dc22

                                                                2010007736

A catalogue record for this book is available from the British Library.

Set in 10/12.5 pt Palatino by Aptara® Inc., New Delhi, India

1   2010

Contents

List of Boxes, Figures and Tables		vi
The Authors		viii
Series Foreword		ix
Acknowledgements		xi
Glossary		xii

Introduction   1

1. Interprofessional teamwork – the basics   10

2. Current developments affecting interprofessional teamwork   24

3. Interprofessional teamwork: key concepts and issues   39

4. A conceptual framework for interprofessional teamwork   57

5. Using theory to better understand interprofessional teamwork   77

6. Interprofessional teamwork interventions   91

7. Evaluating interprofessional teamwork   105

8. Synthesising studies of interprofessional teamwork   121

9. Ways forward   137

References   144
Appendices   164
Index   189

List of Boxes, Figures and Tables

Boxes

1.1. Building teamwork in a rural Australian community   13
1.2. The Brazilian Family Health Team Programme   14
1.3. The family health team initiative in Canada   15
1.4. The STRETCH Project in South Africa   16
1.5. UK-based interprofessional teamwork in maternity care   17
1.6. The Magnet Hospital initiative in the US   18
2.1. Operating room team members' perceptions of error   26
2.2. The development of collaborative patient-centred practice in Canada   27
2.3. A recently funded study on interprofessional teamwork in stroke care   32
2.4. IT and teamwork   34
3.1. The influence of team tasks on teamwork   41
3.2. An example of interprofessional teamwork   45
3.3. An example of interprofessional collaboration   46
3.4. An example of interprofessional coordination   46
3.5. An example of an interprofessional network   47
3.6. An adaptive interprofessional team   47
3.7. A comparison of teamwork based in private and public funded settings   51
4.1. Interprofessional teamwork and hierarchy   59
4.2. How routines and spatial issues affect teamwork   66
4.3. The role of organisational support in teamwork   70
4.4. An insight into how contextual factors can affect teamwork   73
5.1. The use of Marris's psychodynamic theory on loss and change   81
5.2. The use of Tajfel and Turner's social identity theory   82
5.3. The use of a sociological perspective – Goffman's interactionist approach   84
5.4. The use of Engeström's activity theory in medical wards   85
5.5. The use the professionalisation approach to understand medical sports teams   87

5.6. The use of Foucauldian theory in primary care teams   89
6.1. Interprofessional team training intervention   93
6.2. A team communication intervention   95
6.3. An integrated care pathway intervention   97
6.4. Introducing a new role into primary care   98
6.5. A multifaceted teamwork intervention based in general medicine 101
6.6. An example of consultant-led intervention   104
7.1. Examples of formative and summative evaluations   109
7.2. Uses of local knowledge in understanding or improving
       teamworking   111
7.3. An example of qualitative study used to develop an intervention 115
7.4. A qualitative study of intervention implementation processes   116
7.5. A mixed methods study   119
8.1. Factors which limited the effects of teamwork interventions   134
8.2. Implications for the future design of teamwork interventions   136

Figures

3.1. Differing forms of interprofessional work   44
4.1. A framework for understanding interprofessional teamwork   58

Tables

3.1. Synthesising some elements of teamwork   41
3.2. Making sense of different teamwork typologies   48
3.3. Summary of factors influencing team performance   50
5.1. Social science theories that aid better understanding of
       interprofessional teamwork   79
6.1. Summarising interprofessional team interventions   102
7.1. Teamwork evaluation questions for different teamwork activities 110
8.1. Overview of the key features of the included interprofessional
       studies   124
8.2. Main findings from the three studies   126

The Authors

Scott Reeves is a sociologist and a Scientist at the Keenan Research Centre, Li Ka Shing Knowledge Institute of St Michael's Hospital and the Wilson Centre, University Health Network, Toronto, Canada. He is also the Director of Research, Centre for Faculty Development, St. Michael's Hospital, and an Associate Professor in the Department of Psychiatry at the University of Toronto and Editor-in-Chief of the *Journal of Interprofessional Care.*

Simon Lewin trained as a physician and now works as a social scientist and health service researcher. He holds research positions in the Norwegian Knowledge Centre for the Health Services and in the Health Systems Research Unit of Medical Research Council of South Africa, where his work is focused largely on mixed method implementation research in low- and middle-income countries. He is also an editor for the Cochrane Consumers and Communication Review Group and the Cochrane Effective Practice and Organisation of Care Review Group.

Sherry Espin is a registered nurse and an Associate Professor in the Daphne Cockwell School of Nursing, Ryerson University, Toronto. She previously held several positions in perioperative clinical practice and education. She currently teaches in the post diploma and graduate programmes at Ryerson University, with an emphasis on qualitative research, interprofessional education and collaboration, current issues and nursing practice courses.

Merrick Zwarenstein is a physician and a health services researcher. He is a Senior Scientist at the Sunnybrook Research Institute and at the Institute for Clinical Evaluative Sciences, and an Associate Professor in the Department of Health Policy Management and Evaluation at the University of Toronto.

Series Foreword

Promoting partnership for health

Such is the faith in the efficacy of teamwork between professions in health and social care that it is in danger of being reified as a self-evident virtue in need of neither justification nor critical review.

Challenging complacency, Scott Reeves and his co-authors subject interprofessional teamwork to critical scrutiny, mindful throughout of their obligation to chart ways through the labyrinth of problems. Sceptical about facile solutions imported from other working worlds, they drive home the need for critical investigation, generated within health and social care. Grounding arguments in evidence, they put a premium on systematic and rigorous evaluation, contributing unstintingly from their own wealth of experience. Cautioning against reliance on any one theory or discipline, they complement perspectives from dynamic and social psychology, with which readers may be more familiar, with others from sociology, with which they may be less familiar. Conceptualising teamwork, they construct a robust and user-friendly framework which promises to find an enduring place in the understanding of collaboration between professions.

The outcome is a groundbreaking contribution to the teamwork literature and a noteworthy addition to the Wiley/CAIPE series. Packed with implications for policy makers, service managers and practising professionals as much as teachers, students and researchers, the book complements others in the series, especially Meads and Ashcroft (2005), by introducing a much-needed critique of teamwork into the politics and practice of collaboration, and Glasby and Dickinson (2009), by reminding us that integrated services, however well conceived, can only be as good as the teamwork between the people entrusted with their implementation.

The book also provides a much-needed resource to help remedy the shortfall in teamwork teaching and learning on professional and interprofessional courses in health and social care (see Barr *et al.*, 2005; Freeth *et al.*, 2005). Teachers and students will find this book indispensable. It is being published concurrently with another in the series by Mick McKeown and colleagues (2010) which puts collaboration with service users and carers at the heart of not only health and social care practice but also education.

Partnership for health – the catchphrase which we chose for this series – has many meanings to explore from many angles.

Hugh Barr
Series Editor
Emeritus Professor of Interprofessional Education
University of Westminster, UK

The books in the series

Barr H, Koppel I, Reeves S, Hammick M & Freeth D (2005) *Effective Interprofessional Education: Argument, Assumption and Evidence*. Blackwell Publishing, Oxford.

Freeth D, Hammick M, Reeves S, Koppel I & Barr H (2005) *Effective Interprofessional Education: Development, Delivery and Evaluation*. Blackwell Publishing, Oxford.

Glasby J & Dickinson H (2009) *International Perspectives on Health and Social Care*. Wiley-Blackwell, Oxford.

McKeown M, Malihi-Shoja L & Downe S with the Comensus Writing Collective (2010) *Service User and Carer Involvement in Education for Health and Social Care*. Wiley-Blackwell, Oxford.

Meads G & Ashcroft J with Barr H, Scott R & Wild A (2005) *The Case for Collaboration in Health and Social Care*. Blackwell Publishing, Oxford.

Reeves S, Lewin S, Espin S & Zwarenstein M (2010) *Interprofessional Teamwork for Health and Social Care*. Wiley-Blackwell, Oxford.

Acknowledgements

We would like to acknowledge the help of Ilona Abramovich and Abigail Wickson Griffiths for their work in providing a range of materials for the book; and Joanne Goldman for her critical feedback on an earlier draft of the text.

We are also very grateful for the support of our colleagues who were very generous in offering materials for the book and/or providing critical feedback on the contents of draft chapters – in alphabetical order – Anne Biringer, Simon Carmel, Philip Clark, Shelley Cohen Konrad, Signe Flottorp, John Gilbert, Brigid Gillespie, Pippa Hall, Ruth Harris, Gillian Hewitt, Valerie Iles, Chris Kenaszchuk, Byrony Lamb, Tony Leiba, Jill Maben, Pat Mayers, Mary McAllister, Filomena Meffe, Patricia Parra, Madeline Schmitt, Brian Simmons, Sarah Sims, Julian Smith, Kerry Uebel, Elisabeth Willumsen and Charmaine Zankowicz.

We would also like to acknowledge the support of our various institutions in the writing of this book.

Lastly, but importantly, we would like thank all our partners and families who supported us while we worked on the text. In particular, Scott would like to express a special note of thanks to Ruth for her continued support and for her (extreme) patience during the writing of this book; he would also like to thank William, Ewan and Joshua for their patience. Simon would like to thank his partner, Simon G, for his support on this and many other endeavours.

Glossary

Appreciative inquiry is a method, often employed by consultants, which encourages individuals to adopt a positive approach in managing organisational change. This method has, however, been criticised for its lack of critical analysis.

Asynchronous communication takes place between individuals who do not meet in the same physical space at the same time. Often technology such as emails or electronic messages boards is used for this type of communication.

Benchmark statements outline expectations about standards on programmes such as *interprofessional education* (see below). They define what is expected from an individual in terms of the abilities and skills they should achieve when completing a programme of study.

Case management is an approach which involves a single practitioner – usually a nurse or a social worker – who takes the responsibility for and coordination of patient care by liaison and collaboration with other health and social care professions.

Collaboration is an active and ongoing partnership, often between people from diverse backgrounds, who work together to solve problems or provide services.

Collaborative patient-centred practice is a type of arrangement designed to promote the participation of patients and their families within a context of collaborative practice.

Computer conferencing is an audio-visual conference where communication takes place via computers. This type of conference can be held on an *asynchronous* (see above) or *synchronous* (see below) basis.

Continuous quality improvement (CQI) see *quality improvement*.

Crew resource management (CRM) is an approach which emerged from the airline industry which aimed to improve safety among airline crews by providing explicit written procedures which cover a range of potential situations and problems they may encounter.

Direct teamwork interventions aim to improve teamwork by the use of a direct form of action, such as *interprofessional education* (see below). They contrast with *indirect teamwork interventions* (see below).

Epistemology refers to an individual's beliefs about the nature of knowledge and how it is generated. It is also a discipline in philosophy in which individuals study the nature of knowledge.

Ethnography is a methodology that aims to understand the meanings and behaviours associated with the membership of teams, groups and organisations through the collection of observational and interview data.

Evaluation refers to the systematic gathering and interpretation of evidence enabling judgement of effectiveness and value, and promoting improvement. Evaluations can have both *formative* (see below) and/or *summative* (see below) strands.

Expert patient programmes are lay-led self-management initiatives that have been developed for people living with long-term chronic health conditions.

Formative evaluation is usually undertaken during the development of interventions, programmes and initiatives. Its aim is to understand the nature of the early processes, outcomes and impact of activities in order to improve them.

Indirect teamwork interventions usually aim to improve the delivery of care, by use of teamwork. Although teams are involved in this type of intervention, its aim is not to explicitly improve teamwork.

Integrated care pathways are interventions in which the activities involved in a patient's care trajectory are specified along a certain trajectory time period; also called 'critical pathways', 'collaborative care plans' and 'multidisciplinary action plans'.

Interactionism is a sociological theory which regards the social world as one which is primarily constructed through an individual's interactions with others.

Interdisciplinary teamwork relates to the collaborative efforts undertaken by individuals from different disciplines such as psychology, anthropology, economics, geography, political science and computer science.

Interpretivism is a philosophy which is based on the notion that the social world is interpreted by individuals in their thoughts and language. The social world is constructed through individuals' actions, interactions and the meanings they attach to these activities. Qualitative research methods (interviews and observations) are located within an interpretivist approach.

Interprofessional collaboration is a type of interprofessional work which involves different health and social care professions who regularly come together to solve problems or provide services.

Interprofessional coordination is a type of work, similar to *interprofessional collaboration* (see above) as it involves different health and social care professions. It differs as it is a 'looser' form of working arrangement whereby interprofessional communication and discussion may be less frequent.

Interprofessional education occurs when members (or students) of two or more health and/or social care professions engage in interactive learning activities to improve collaboration and/or the delivery of care.

Interprofessional interventions involve two or more health and social care professions who learn and/or work together to improve their approach to *collaboration* (see above).

Interprofessional networks are loosely organised groups of individuals from different health and social care professions, who meet and work together on a periodic basis.

Interprofessional teamwork is a type of work which involves different health and/or social professions who share a team identity and work closely together in an integrated and interdependent manner to solve problems and deliver services.

Intraprofessional is a term which describes any activity which is undertaken by individuals within the same profession.

Kaizen see *quality improvement*.

Lean methodology see *quality improvement*.

Meta-ethnography is a type of literature review (see below) which searches, analyses and synthesises qualitative research studies to understand the nature of a specific topic.

Mixed methods study is an empirical approach which employs both qualitative (e.g. interviews) and quantitative (e.g. surveys) methods of inquiry.

Multidisciplinary teamwork is an approach like *interprofessional teamwork* (see above), but differs as the team members are composed from different academic disciplines (psychology, sociology, mathematics) rather than from different professions such as medicine, nursing and social work.

Multifaceted intervention is an intervention which consists of different but linked strands of activity designed to meet a common goal, such as the improvement of teamwork.

Paradigms refer to the underpinning knowledge which forms and shapes all of the natural science (e.g. physics, chemistry) and social science (e.g. sociology, economics) disciplines.

Patient-centred care is an approach to delivering care which advocates that patients and their relatives are located at the centre of the care-giving process. It emerged in response to concerns that care was too professionally oriented.

Patriarchy is a term which refers to the organisation of social relations whereby men are dominant and control, in large part, the socio-economic and political resources of a society.

Positivism is a philosophy which holds that knowledge is generated through the phenomena we physically experience. The purpose of positivistic science is therefore to observe and measure, usually by quantitative (numeric, statistics-based) methods, those things we physically experience.

Professionalisation is a sociological approach which has been developed to help understand the processes related to the historical development of different health and social care professions.

Quality circles see *quality improvement*.

Quality improvement is an approach based on a manufacturing philosophy and set of methods for reducing time from customer order to product delivery, costing less, taking less space and improving quality. Also called CQI (continuous quality improvement), Kaizen, Lean Methodology, Quality Circles, Six Sigma and TQM (total quality management).

Randomised trial is a test of the efficacy of an intervention which seeks to control for intervening variables by randomly allocating subjects into either an intervention group or a control group. It may be blind, double blind or triple blind depending upon whether subjects, researchers or practitioners have knowledge of the group (intervention or control) to which a subject is allocated.

Reflexivity is a research technique which recognises how the researchers' own influences, generated from a number of sources (e.g. gender, ethnic background, social status) may affect their scholarly work.

Reviews are undertaken to synthesise the findings generated from a number of individual studies. Reviews can be narrative (descriptive), critical or *systematic* (see below).

Scoping review is a type of *review* (see above) which is exploratory in nature and aims to generate an initial insight into the nature of evidence related to a particular topic. Often, scoping reviews are completed before *systematic reviews* (see below) are undertaken.

Six sigma see *quality improvement*.

Summative evaluation aims to judge the success of interventions, programmes and initiatives in relation to their 'final' outcome(s) and impact. This type of evaluation is usually undertaken to account for resources and also to inform future planning.

Synchronous communication takes place between individuals in 'real time' in meetings or by use of the telephone or electronic (computer-based) conferencing.

Systematic review is a type of review which aims to identify, synthesise and appraise all the high-quality research evidence related to a particular topic.

Total quality management (TQM) see *quality improvement*.

Triangulation is a research technique in which researchers compare the findings of different methods (interviews, surveys), theories and/or perspectives of different people to generate more comprehensive insights.

Uniprofessional see *intraprofessional*.

Validity refers to the degree to which a study accurately reflects the phenomena that the researcher is attempting to investigate/measure.

Videoconferencing is a type of electronic conferencing which uses video to support simultaneous interaction between individuals.

Wikipedia is an online resource which provides information on a range of subjects (see: http://www.wikipedia.org/).

Introduction

Over the past 25 years, attention has been placed increasingly on how interprofessional teams can improve professional relationships, collaboration and quality of care. As a result, improved teamwork is a near-universal aspiration of health and social care practitioners, managers and organisations. Indeed, it is often assumed that teamwork is *the* way in which professional relations should be managed and care should be delivered. The topic has received a significant amount of attention from researchers and policy makers, and has been described and discussed in a range of books, papers and reports. However, this literature still only provides a relatively limited understanding of its complex nature.

For us, the inadequate progress in developing a deeper understanding of teamwork is, in part, a result of many teamwork texts and papers being based on *a priori* assumption that teams are a 'good thing', and that they offer a solution to alleviating a number of the ills of health and social care systems. While there is an intuitive appeal in this view, its consequence is that few authors have drilled down to the empirical, conceptual and theoretical bedrock upon which teamwork rests.

In this book we aim to cut through the rhetoric currently associated with interprofessional teams to examine, in some depth, the complex array of elements, factors and issues which affect the ways in which professionals work together. We explore a range of concepts and theories which help to understand interprofessional teamwork; examine the evidence on the effects of interventions to promote teamworking; and discuss approaches to its evaluation.

Why interprofessional teamwork?

Patients, clients and service users frequently have conditions that have multiple causes and require multiple treatments from a range of health and social care professions with different skills and expertise. As it is unusual for one profession to deliver a complete episode of care in isolation, good quality care depends upon professions working together in interprofessional teams. Indeed, Rafferty *et al.* (2001, p. 33) argued that 'the value of teamwork has an intuitive appeal'. Indeed, teamwork is regarded by many stakeholders as key to the delivery of effective care systems. For example, a recent document published by the Canadian Health Services Research Foundation (2006, p. 1) states:

> A healthcare system that supports effective teamwork can improve the quality of patient care, enhance patient safety, and reduce workloads that cause burnout among healthcare professionals.

In general, when a team works 'well', it does so because every member has a role. Every member not only knows and executes their own role with great skill and creativity, they also know the responsibilities and activities of every other role on the team, as well as having an understanding of the personal nuances that each individual brings to their role. This complicated range of elements needs to simultaneously occur if the team is to function in an effective manner. As a result, such a description tends only to cover a small number of health and social care teams. Indeed, this view represents an *ideal* type towards which teams in health and social care work, not a description of how they routinely function. This book is inspired by the ideal. Importantly, it aims at closing the gap between that ideal and the reality.

Why read this book?

This book is addressed to health and social care providers, students, managers, policy makers, researchers and educators as well as the consumers of their services. Below are some reasons why this book should be read:

- It aims to provide a scholarly, yet accessible text that explores and critiques key issues, concepts, interventions, theories and evidence regarding teamwork. Our overall intention is to offer readers with a critical assessment of the benefits and limitations of teamworking, evaluating the evidence for different approaches and identifying where evidence still needs to be gathered to inform practice.
- The book does not promote one specific approach to understanding teamwork but draws upon a wide range of approaches and attempts to synthesise their key lessons to help inform health and social care providers, educators and researchers.
- The book draws together evidence and practice from a wide range of settings, in low-, middle- and high-income countries and examines the similarities and differences in teamworking across these different contexts.
- It aims to provide evidence and guidance for those who wish to commission, design, develop and implement interprofessional teamwork interventions to improve collaboration as well as evaluate the effects of their interventions in a comprehensive manner.
- The book contains a set of ideas and approaches (see Appendices) which aim to help readers understand and evaluate the interprofessional teams in which they work in order to enhance their function.

- For patients, clients and service users, the book aims to offer an insight into a range of issues, factors and challenges related to delivering their care in an interprofessional team-based fashion.

Our focus

The book considers interprofessional teamwork across a range of different national contexts. We ourselves have personal experience of teamwork from four different countries – Canada, Norway, South Africa and the UK. Our personal and professional networks expand this reach into numerous other countries, including, Australia, Denmark, Japan, Sweden and the United States.

In addition to examining the differences and similarities between contexts, we consider how interprofessional teamwork operates across a variety of different clinical settings, including general medicine, resuscitation, stroke, rehabilitation, paediatric, geriatric, surgical and community mental health teams.

We also consider interprofessional teamwork issues in relation to the delivery of clinical care, the management of care, diagnostics work and health promotion – wherever interprofessional teamwork occurs in health and social care. The book therefore spans a range of contexts in which professionals work in close proximity with more or less continuous communication, to those working at a distance, who need only to communicate episodically.

When relevant, we compare the experiences of health and social care teams with those from industry, drawing on the wider literature about teams to broaden our understanding of how interprofessional teams operate.

Our focus is inclusive. We employ a definition of team which not only includes the usual professional 'suspects' such as medicine, nursing, occupational therapy, physiotherapy and social work but also draws upon the perspectives of administrators, managers, support staff, health care assistants as well as patients and their carers/relatives. We also intend to assess how a wide range of professional, organisational and structural factors interplay within an interprofessional team-based context.

Overall, the book aims to enrich readers, understanding of interprofessional teamwork, exploring how teamwork connects with other interprofessional activities such as patient safety and interprofessional education. It also aims to provide a set of ideas and approaches aimed to help develop, implement, evaluate and better understand teamwork.

Conceptual considerations

We view interprofessional teamwork as an activity which is founded upon a range of key dimensions including:

- Clear goals (the primary goal being effective patient/client care)
- Shared team identity
- Shared commitment
- Clear team roles and responsibilities
- Interdependence between team members
- Integration between work practices.

While other authors have employed the terms 'interprofessional teamwork' and 'interprofessional collaboration' interchangeably, we view teamwork as a specific type of work. For example, we see collaboration as a broad activity whereby two or more people interact to advance some form of endeavour – in health and social care this is usually to improve the delivery of patient/client care. Teamwork, on the other hand, is a more focused activity. In Chapter 3 we introduce the *contingency* approach to interprofessional work – an approach which encourages the 'matching' of a particular type of interprofessional work (teamwork, collaboration, coordination and networking) depending upon local care needs and demands.

Our approach to interprofessional teamwork is, in many ways, an ideal of what it *could be*, not necessarily what currently *is*. As noted above, such an ideal of teamwork inspired this book. Nevertheless, teams function in the *real world*, and as a result they are affected by a 'cocktail' of individual, professional, organisational, educational and structural factors which can impede their performance and function.

Indeed, in attempting to uncover and study the ingredients of this cocktail, we have drawn on a number of sources (the teamwork literature, our own academic work, our personal and clinical experiences as well as conversations with colleagues). These sources have helped develop an interprofessional framework which consists of a number of different factors which we have clustered together into the following four domains:

- *Relational*: Factors linked to how interprofessional relations are influenced. The focus of this domain is upon understanding how issues such as power, hierarchy, leadership and membership influence team function (or dysfunction).
- *Processual*: Aspects linked to understanding how the actual working practices undertaken by team members affect teamwork. The focus of this domain is on exploring how, for example, time, space and task complexity affect teamwork.
- *Organisational*: The local environment in which the interprofessional team operates. The focus of this domain is upon understanding organisational structures in which the team is based and the commitment/support of the organisation.
- *Contextual*: The broad cultural, political, social, economic landscape in which the team is located. The focus of this domain is upon understanding how structural influences can affect interprofessional teamwork.

We expand this framework in Chapter 4, describing the various factors and discussing their implications for working in an interprofessional team. In addition, we employ the framework in a number of other chapters to provide a narrative thread for the book as well as help understand the complex and interlinked nature of interprofessional teamwork across various contextual and care settings.

Our stance

In writing this book we have thought very carefully about its stance. Below is an outline the underlying assumptions and ideas we share as co-authors, which have had an influence on producing this text.

Critical

While we value positive applications of interprofessional teamwork to the delivery of care, we are trained as researchers to think critically. Rather than simply accepting the largely positive assumptions, ideas and arguments about interprofessional teamwork, we *problematise* them. We examine, question and probe the current rhetoric about interprofessional teamwork to provide a critical account of the potential challenges associated with this approach.

Pluralistic

We employ a pluralistic approach to our understanding of teamwork from our differing academic, professional and disciplinary lenses – sociological, nursing, epidemiological and medical – which we value in providing a range of (sometimes contrasting) interpretations or views of teamwork. Rather than privileging one dominant view, we employ these different perspectives in a pluralistic manner to help paint a more balanced, comprehensive and detailed picture of interprofessional teamwork.

Pragmatic

As researchers involved in undertaking research in the real world, we are pragmatic in our approach. While we value experiential knowledge, as an initial step for building evidence, we are directed towards evidence-based approaches to interprofessional teamwork – where they exist. As we noted above, we are critical, so we critique the quality of evidence reported in journals, reports, book chapters and textbooks. We do this in order to provide a *realistic* account of its impact – positive, neutral or negative.

Reflexive

We all value reflexivity in our academic work. We therefore try to be reflexive about our own experiences of interprofessional teamwork and its evaluation. For example, SE worked for many years as an operating theatre nurse and has subsequently evaluated teamwork in this setting. In the book she draws upon how her clinical experiences shaped her views of teamworking and informed the questions she later asked in her research.

Optimistic

We believe that the complexity of health and social care have compelled the creation of multiple professions, who need to work together to address patient problems. We think this increasing proliferation of professions and increasingly dense set of shared tasks irreversibly point to a future in which the health and social care systems are built entirely on teamwork and collaboration. We believe this is positive, as it brings to bear a broader range of skills, deeper deliberations and a more appropriate range of choices in facing each problem. Therefore, despite our critical perspective, we remain optimistic about the future of interprofessional teamwork.

Introducing the team

We are an interprofessional and interdisciplinary team of researchers representing medicine, nursing, sociology, epidemiology, health services and health professions education research. We have worked in a variety of interprofessional teams during our careers based in clinical and academic settings. We bring these experiences to the book to provide as rich a text as possible. We also bring findings from our collective and collaborative studies of interprofessional teams in high-, low- and middle-income countries, as well as insights based on numerous projects which have aimed to develop and implement teamwork interventions.

Some further information about each of us:

SR: I am a sociologist who has worked as a researcher in health services and health professions education for nearly 15 years in both the UK and in Canada. My main research interests focus on exploring and evaluating the processes and outcomes related to interprofessional education and practice (both in terms of interprofessional teamwork and collaboration). Methodologically, I am primarily an ethnographic researcher, although I do often stray into other methodological areas such as mixed methods research and systematic review. Theoretically, I am most influenced by the sociological work of Anselm Strauss and Erving Goffman.

SL: I am a physician and social scientist working as a health services researcher mainly in low- and middle-income country settings. My current work is largely within the field of implementation research, including the development and evaluation of strategies for changing professional practice and the organisation of care within primary care teams and the roles of lay providers within health systems. My methodological interests are in ways of drawing together outcome and process findings in the context of randomised controlled trials; systematic reviews of complex interventions; and methods for synthesising the findings of qualitative studies.

SE: I am a nurse, teacher and researcher. My PhD thesis focused on the diversity of interprofessional team members' perspectives on error, error disclosure and reporting as well as patients' perceptions of these issues. My current programme of research seeks to theorise how professionals on the health care team interact with one another in the context of perceived errors of care, in settings such as the intensive care unit, the operating room and the medical inpatient ward.

MZ: I am a physician, with experience in family medicine and ambulatory chronic disease care, but for many years now I have been exclusively a researcher in these fields. My research focuses on strategies for achieving evidence-based care in health systems, drawing on educational and social techniques for implementation. Methodologically, my expertise is in pragmatic randomised trials of complex interventions, often in collaboration with colleagues from other professions and disciplines (i.e. economists, qualitative researchers).

Outline

The book is divided into nine chapters, which take the reader on a journey that covers salient issues, concepts, interventions, studies and theories related to interprofessional teamwork.

Chapters

In Chapter 1 we set the scene by outlining some common issues which underpin interprofessional teamwork. We also discuss some of the key reasons behind the need for this type of interprofessional approach as well as outlining the historical development related to the emergence of teamwork across a range of different countries and clinical contexts.

We continue the scene setting in Chapter 2 as we discuss the range of current developments which are contributing to the growth in interprofessional teams and teamwork around the globe, including health care economics, human resource factors, educational developments, changes in the health care professions and shifting patient demographics.

In Chapter 3 we identify and discuss the range of key concepts and typologies related to interprofessional teams and teamwork. Specifically, we focus on the various concepts related to differing types of team structures, roles and team processes. We also explore and critique the applicability of teamwork approaches rooted in other settings (e.g. crew resource management) and adopted in health and social care. We also introduce our *contingency approach* to interprofessional work, one which assesses local need before employing one of four different ways of working together – teamwork, collaboration, coordination and networking.

In Chapter 4 we present our framework of interprofessional teamwork which contains a number of factors that we have clustered together in four domains – relational, processual, organisational and contextual. Through the use of this framework, we examine the various factors, such as professional power, gender, organisational support and information technology that can affect the way in which members of interprofessional teams work together.

In Chapter 5 we explore and compare a range of different but complementary social science theories which help illuminate our understanding of interprofessional teamwork. Using our framework, we present, discuss and apply these theories to the relational, processual, organisational and contextual factors related to interprofessional teamwork.

In Chapter 6 we describe and critique a range of interprofessional interventions (e.g. interprofessional education, quality improvement, team-based communication) designed to help improve interprofessional teamwork and the delivery of care. We employ our framework to delineate and discuss the nature of these different interprofessional interventions.

In Chapter 7 we provide a description of the various methodological approaches (quantitative, qualitative and mixed methods) taken to evaluate interprofessional teamwork and build its empirical base. We discuss the relative strengths and limitations of each approach as well as provide examples of different types of teamwork evaluation.

In Chapter 8 we synthesise research which we have been undertaking over the past 15 years on teamwork and collaboration in Canada, South Africa and the UK. We go on to embed this work in the wider literature to offer implications related to effective interprofessional team function.

In Chapter 9 we draw together the key threads of the book. We both distil the core elements of this text and offer ideas on future directions for interprofessional teamwork intervention and evaluation.

Appendices

We also present a range of interprofessional teamwork resources in the form of five appendices which are designed to provide a variety of ideas on the planning, designing, implementing and evaluation of teamwork activities.

Summaries, reflections and experiences

To broaden the perspective of the book, throughout the chapters we have offered the following:

- Summaries of published interprofessional teamwork studies
- Reflections from interprofessional 'gurus' from Canada, the UK and the US who offer personal accounts of teamwork in the past 30 years as well as ideas for the future of teamwork

- Experiences from a range of professionals from Australia, Norway, South Africa, the UK and the US, who have worked within different interprofessional health and social care teams.

Some notes on terminology

As noted above, we take an inclusive view on team membership. For us, an interprofessional team can include those professions most often associated with health care delivery, such as nursing, medicine, occupational therapy and social work, but also a range of other groups including health support workers, managers, assistants who all need to collaborate in the delivery of care.

This is a book about interprofessional teamwork. Its focus, therefore, is upon those individuals – from different professions – who interact and work together to deliver health and social care. This is not a book on *interdisciplinary* teamwork which we see as a broader activity which can involve the interaction of individuals from different disciplines such as psychology, anthropology, economics, political science and computer science for a range of purposes. As we discuss later in the book, the teamwork literature can be confusing as authors employ a range of terms such as interdisciplinary, multidisciplinary, multiprofessional and transprofessional. However, we have carefully assessed the materials we have used in the book to only include those which have a focus on 'interprofessional teamwork', despite their labelling.

Although we are very aware of the sensitivities about the use of the term 'patient' especially when referring to healthy individuals who receive health and social care services, for simplicity we employ this term to cover the range of other descriptions (e.g. client, service user, consumer).

1 Interprofessional teamwork – the basics

Introduction

In this chapter we outline some of the 'basics' of interprofessional teamwork. In doing so, we describe a range of conceptual, political, historical and experiential elements related to the ways in which teams function. Our focus here is deliberately wide – to provide readers with an initial 'taste' of some of the elements that will be discussed in more depth in subsequent chapters. First, we outline a number of key dimensions of interprofessional teamwork. We then go on to explain why interprofessional teamwork is regarded as central to addressing a wide spectrum of health and social care service delivery problems. Next, we trace the emergence of interprofessional teamwork over the past 100 years, drawing on examples from a number of different countries and clinical contexts. To provide insights into contemporary teamwork issues, we go on to present direct accounts of professionals' experiences of interprofessional teamwork in health and social care settings in a range of countries. Finally, we outline a range of implications for interprofessional teamwork.

Key dimensions of interprofessional teamwork

As noted in the Introduction, we view interprofessional teamwork as an activity which is based on a number of key dimensions. These include: clear team goals; a shared team identity; shared team commitment; role clarity; interdependence; and integration between team members. Our perspective on the important dimensions of teamworking is similar to those of our colleagues (e.g. Øvretveit, 1993; Meerabeau and Page, 1999; Onyett, 2003; Jelphs and Dickenson, 2008), which we introduce in later chapters.

Drawing on a study of primary care teams, West and Slater (1996) have usefully extended our thinking about the key dimensions of interprofessional teamwork. They found that team members viewed a number of additional elements of teamwork as being important, including:

- Democratic approaches
- Efforts to breakdown stereotypes and barriers
- Regular time to develop teamworking away from practice
- Good communication
- A single shared work location
- Mutual role understanding
- The development of joint protocols, training and work practices
- Agreed practice priorities across professional boundaries
- Regular and effective team meetings
- Team members valuing and respecting each other
- Good performance management.

Currently, however, we do not have a strong body of high quality, empirical evidence that confirms how these different elements – individually or collectively – affect interprofessional teamwork. Nevertheless, the dimensions listed above provide a useful reminder of the complex and multifaceted nature of this type of work. Accounts from the literature of the difficulties experienced in implementing interprofessional teamwork further highlight this complexity (e.g. Cott, 1998; Skjørshammer, 2001; Allen, 2002; Reeves *et al.*, 2009c). Writing from a UK perspective, the Audit Commission (1992, p. 20) has pointed out that:

> Separate lines of control, different payment systems leading to suspicion over motives, diverse objectives, professional barriers and perceived inequalities in status, all play a part in limiting the potential of multiprofessional, multi-agency teamwork [. . .]. For those working under such circumstances efficient teamwork remains elusive.

In later chapters we investigate the complex nature of interprofessional teamwork, and explore why individuals can (and often do) experience difficulties when working as members of an interprofessional team.

Growing support for interprofessional teamwork

There has been a growing support for the use of interprofessional teamwork across health and social care settings. This support can be seen in the numerous papers and documents which argue that interprofessional teamwork is an essential ingredient for reducing duplication of effort, improving coordination, enhancing safety and, therefore, delivering high quality care (e.g. Shaw, 1970; Gregson *et al.*, 1991; Farrell *et al.*, 2001; Schmitt, 2001; Onyett, 2003). Eichhorn (1974, p. 6) offers an early argument for why interprofessional teams are needed in the delivery of care:

> Health [and social care] problems have become defined in complex and multi-faceted terms. Health organisations have discovered it is necessary to have the information and skills of many disciplines in order to develop valid solutions and deliver comprehensive care to individuals and families.

This view was reiterated more recently by Firth-Cozens (1998, p. 3) who has argued that:

Teamworking is seen as a way to tackle the potential fragmentation of care; a means to widen skills; an essential part of the need to consider the complexity of modern care; and a way to generally improve quality for the patient.

Similar sentiments can be found in a range of national government policies (e.g. Department of Health, 1997; Health Council of Canada, 2009), as well as in the documents and policies of professional regulatory bodies (e.g. General Medical Council, 2001; Association of American Medical Colleges, 2009) and international agencies (e.g. World Health Organization, 1988). As the National Health Service Management Executive (1993) in the UK stated:

The best and most cost-effective outcomes for patients and clients are achieved when professionals work together, learn together, engage in clinical audit of outcomes together, and generate innovation to ensure progress in practice and service. (Paragraph 4.3)

Repeated arguments for interprofessional teamwork as well as the policy level calls for its implementation have resulted in an expansion of teamwork activities across the globe. Indeed, the range of different countries reporting interprofessional teamwork activities has rapidly increased in recent years. In addition to countries with a long track record of teamwork initiatives, such as Australia, Canada, the UK and the US, a number of other countries, including Brazil (Peres *et al.*, 2006), China (Lee, 2003), New Zealand (Pullon *et al.*, 2009), Spain (Goñi, 1999), Sweden (Kvarnström, 2008) and The Gambia (Conn *et al.*, 1996), are also reporting the use of interprofessional teamwork across a number of clinical contexts. We provide more detail on the nature of these different teamwork initiatives in the next section where we describe and discuss the emergence of interprofessional teamwork across a number of continents.

The emergence of teamwork

In this part of the chapter we offer a number of vignettes on the development of teamwork from different settings. Our aim is to illustrate how teamwork activities have evolved over time in different contexts and how it has come to the forefront of health and social care policymaking in the following six countries – Australia, Brazil, Canada, South Africa, the UK and the US.

Australia

National and state government policy directives in Australia have repeatedly noted that collaboration is a key element in improving service delivery (e.g. Australian Government, 2009). Policies such as the *Enhanced Primary Care and Medication* initiative aim to encourage the delivery of more effective care through interprofessional teamwork (McNair *et al.*, 2001). The importance of interprofessional teams in providing primary care services is therefore increasingly recognised. However, it has been noted that progress has been restricted by traditional funding arrangements which emphasise parallel working and poor integration of professions. Efforts are currently focused on strengthening collaboration between GPs, nurses, midwives, therapists, pharmacists and dentists (Australian Government, 2008). One particular ongoing challenge is the provision of health and social care in rural areas which demands a very particular interprofessional team approach – see Box 1.1.

Box 1.1 Building teamwork in a rural Australian community.

Fuller *et al.* (2004) describe a qualitative study which involved eliciting the perspectives of 200 local stakeholders about developing a mental health plan in a remote region of South Australia. The authors found that the provision of mental healthcare in this region presented a number of difficult challenges for local health and social care practitioners. Although there was a desire by professionals to collaborate more closely with their colleagues, this appeared to be hindered by a lack of understanding of each other's roles and their respective areas of expertise as well as constraints in service delivery. Problems were particularly evident between GPs, who worked on a fee-for-service basis, and members of community mental health teams, who worked for a fixed salary. The authors suggest that agreements need to be struck between professionals about how they can work together to improve their communication and coordination activities. They also note that community mental health teams need to explore how they might work more collaboratively with other providers, such as housing, ambulance and education services, in order to provide a local integrated mental health service.

Brazil

Harzheim *et al.* (2006) note that the disease burden in Brazil results primarily from chronic diseases in adults, most notably hypertension and diabetes. In order to prevent and manage these diseases, the government has shifted its attention from acute to primary care. In 1995 it launched its *Programa Saúde da Família* (Family Health Programme) which aims to promote the use of an interprofessional team approach in primary care across Brazil. Since its inception, the number of teams has grown – collectively they cover 46% of the Brazilian population (Brazilian Government Ministry of Health, 2004). Box 1.2 provides an account of interprofessional relations in this type of team.

Canada

While Szasz (1969) outlined the need for interprofessional education, collaboration and teamwork in his paper published over 40 years ago, there was little response

---

Box 1.2   The Brazilian Family Health Team Programme.

Peres *et al.* (2006) describe an evaluation of the Brazilian Family Health Team programme in the state capital of Rio de Janeiro. Teams within this programme typically serve 600–1000 families and are generally composed of one family practice physician, one nurse, two auxiliary nurses and four to six community workers (team members who focus on disease prevention and health promotion). A survey of over 200 nurses and physicians' views of their approach to collaborative care was conducted following their attendance at a government-funded team training initiative. On the whole, the nurses and physicians reported that they worked in a more collaborative manner, particularly during their weekly team meetings. These meetings focused on shared decision-making about administrative issues, reading and discussing of scientific issues or debate of selected cases, discussion of the weekly team plan and communication of recent developments to the whole team. It was also reported that team members, through their shared work, were increasingly adopting a number of shared values about delivering care in an interprofessional manner.

---

from the Canadian government until the early 1990s. A key initiative, *Collaboration for Prevention*, encouraged health care organisations to implement several projects demonstrating how health care teams could work together and involve patients in decision-making. Building upon this work, the federal government (Health Canada) announced in 2000 that $800m would be distributed through provincial and territorial agreements to support primary care providers develop collaborative approaches. Health Canada also recently launched a Pan-Canadian health human resources strategy to facilitate and support the implementation of an *Interprofessional Education for Collaborative Patient-Centred Practice* initiative across health and social care sectors (see Chapter 2). This followed recommendations in both the Romanow Report (2002) and the First Ministers' Accord (Health Canada, 2003) on reforming the health and education systems to become more collaborative and responsive to patient needs. Box 1.3 outlines a recent initiative aimed at improving patient care through the development of interprofessional primary care teams in one of Canada's largest provinces.

South Africa

The implementation of a district health system in South Africa in the 1990s resulted in a stronger emphasis on primary health care and an enhanced role for teamworking in primary care (South African Department of Health, 2001). Professionals are increasingly expected to collaborate in managing district health services and there is greater discussion of how professional and non-professional providers, such as lay health workers, can better work together in primary health centres. The demand placed on the health system by the HIV/AIDS epidemic has further emphasised the need to use the limited available human resources in the most effective way – a key issue for many low- and middle-income countries. The

> **Box 1.3**   The family health team initiative in Canada.
>
> Meuser *et al.* (2006) describe an Ontario-based initiative which was supported by regional government funding to establish interprofessional family health teams across the province. The initiative marked a departure from the traditional model of uniprofessional physician-based primary care towards one in which a team of health care professionals work together to address the local needs. The authors note that family health teams have a core of physicians, nurse practitioners and nurses, but can also include input from pharmacists and social workers. Team members work collaboratively to ensure that care can be coordinated and delivered in an effective and seamless manner. The overall goals of the family health team initiative include the provision of patient-centred care, improved access to care from a variety of health care professionals, an increased emphasis on chronic disease management, health promotion and disease prevention. The authors note that, to date, over 100 family health teams have been established, each at different stages of implementation. Teams were supported, it was noted, by the Ministry of Health's team guides that cover a range of issues, such as provider compensation, the use of information technology and ideas on establishing clear team roles/responsibilities.

extent to which this rhetoric of teamworking is reflected in changes to policies and practice is unclear, although some novel interventions to promote teamworking in primary care have been implemented. One of these initiatives is discussed further in Box 1.4, which describes a programme to improve teamwork and the delivery of primary care to people living with HIV/AIDS.

The United Kingdom

Interprofessional teamwork has a long history in the evolution of health and social care services in the UK. For Pietroni (1994), two nineteenth-century developments had a significant effect on the nature of modern teamwork. The first was increased government involvement in the delivery of health and social care and a desire within medical profession to delegate a range of their tasks. This, in turn, resulted in the increased involvement of professions, such as nursing and social work, in the delivery of care with physicians. The second was the 'militarisation' of acute care stemming from the Boer and Crimean wars. In response to the challenges of delivering care in the extreme conditions of warfare, medicine (and nursing through the influence of Florence Nightingale) employed the tactics of their military colleagues, including a chain of command, clear roles and hierarchy of decision-making. This approach to organising care was subsequently transported back to civilian life.

Focusing on the period following the formation of the National Health Service (NHS), Leathard (2003a) has traced a number of teamwork developments. She notes that interprofessional teams within hospital settings, particularly in

---

Box 1.4   The STRETCH Project in South Africa.

The STRETCH project – *Streamlining Tasks and Roles to Expand Treatment and Care* for HIV – aims to increase access to anti-retroviral drugs (ARVs) by encouraging nurses to initiate and repeat ARV prescriptions for uncomplicated patients and by integrating HIV and ARV care into primary health care services through interprofessional teamwork (Fairall *et al.*, 2008). Teams were set up at sites where nurses were prescribing ARVs. These teams involved pharmacists and physicians from the treatment sites and nurses from the ARV sites to provide logistics and support for prescribing nurses. Interprofessional teams were also set up with local area managers responsible for health services in that area in order to manage integration of HIV care services into primary care. These teams included pharmacists and nurses. To date, STRETCH has resulted in increased collaboration between physicians, pharmacists and nurses. It functioned less well when the physicians and pharmacists were based in a treatment site at a distance from the nurse-run ARV site. This was particularly difficult when there was a high turnover of pharmacists or physicians, which resulted in a lack of continuity. The teams set up to handle the integration of HIV care into primary care involved people already bringing primary health care services to the community. The services that they were integrating into primary care as part of the STRETCH project included drug readiness training, ARV preparation and monthly ARV care for those patients who had been stabilised at the ARV site. In areas where these teams worked well, they developed a strong sense of collaboration to bring services closer to people while trying to address practical issues such as training, staffing and suitability of facilities to be able to carry out the proposed integration. In some areas these teams did not succeed in working well together, particularly where there were many primary care clinics referring to ARV sites in large urban areas. Vacant management and coordinator posts also resulted in major logistical challenges for the existing ARV services.

---

departments of medicine and surgery, had traditionally formed the core of team-based interactions. However, in the 1970s and 1980s there was an expansion of teamwork into both mental health and primary care settings as a consequence of shifting government policies. More recent developments include, a focus on the use of interprofessional teamwork for patient safety (see Chapter 2) and an increased focus on the role of teamwork within obstetrics (e.g. O'Neill, 2008). Box 1.5 provides an account of a UK study which outlines a recent example of interprofessional teamwork within a maternity care context.

The United States

Like the UK, teamwork in the US has had a long and varied history. An early published example can be found in 1948 by Cherasky who described a *Team*

> **Box 1.5** UK-based interprofessional teamwork in maternity care.
>
> Mackintosh *et al.* (2009) report findings from a qualitative study which explored the notion of 'team situation awareness' – an approach in which team members possess an awareness of their professional and interprofessional roles, tasks and responsibilities. Team situation awareness is noted to be a key factor in the patient safety literature, as it can contribute to safety by promoting effective decision-making, informed by knowledge of the available resources, and linked to the prioritisation and anticipation of tasks. The authors reported findings from a study of the nature of safety within maternity care, which gathered 177 hours of observation focused on teamwork and decision-making across four UK sites. Analysis of the data revealed that three elements were key to facilitating team situation awareness and team coordination – interprofessional handovers, sharing information by use of a whiteboard and a coordinator role (which involved the management of midwifery staff and was usually undertaken by a senior midwife). The authors found that the whiteboard acted as an important 'viewing lens' (p. 52) for physicians. The midwives, in turn, took ownership of the board to add and update clinical information. It was also found that the use of interprofessional handovers and the input of a coordinator were key to distributing information between team members. Collectively, handovers and the coordinator played a third and important additional role in providing *contextualising* information. The authors conclude that context, as well as the interplay between these three facilitating elements, were central components in affecting the quality of teamwork and the level of team situation awareness.

Home Care initiative – an outreach programme based at the Montefoire Hospital in New York State which involved teams of social workers, physicians and nurses (Casto, 1994). Other early developments took place at the University of Washington's Child Health Centre in Seattle which involved the development of interprofessional teams consisting of physicians (paediatricians and psychiatrists), psychologists, nurses and social workers (Casto, 1994). Two notable teamwork developments were the Veterans Administration (VA) hospitals' initiative, which in 1979 provided training programmes to teams working in geriatric settings, and the W.K. Kellogg Foundation, which funded a number of interprofessional team training initiatives in the 1980s. Box 1.6 provides an example of an interprofessional development aimed to improve teamwork between nursing and medicine.

The US has since witnessed a series of other teamwork developments as part of the quality and safety movement (see Chapter 2). Sorbero *et al.* (2008) recently described three current initiatives which have promoted interprofessional teamwork. The first, led by the VA hospitals initiative, involves 20 of its hospitals and was entitled *Transformation of the Operating Room*. This programme implemented

---

Box 1.6   The Magnet Hospital initiative in the US.

The *Magnet Hospital* initiative was nursing-led and promoted interprofessional collaboration and teamwork between nurses, physicians as well as other professionals. This model emerged in the 1980s from a policy study commissioned by the American Academy of Nursing during a time of major nursing shortages (Buchan, 1999). Magnet hospitals were intended to be organisations that attracted well-qualified nurses and offered enhanced nursing roles, job satisfaction and higher than average patient care outcomes (Buchan, 1999). In an evaluation of this initiative, it was found that the Magnet Hospitals were successful in both attracting and maintaining a qualified team of nurses who were willing to engage in new methods to solve problems. This, in turn, led to improved collaboration and teamwork between nurses and other professionals (Kramer and Schmalenberg, 1988).

---

surgical briefings and time-outs to help improve team relations. The second, led by Kaiser Permanente, set out to implement preoperative safety briefing in its 30 hospitals. This was intended to help improve team relations; reduce staff turnover and 'wrong-site' surgeries; and increase the detection of 'near misses'. The third initiative, led by the Institute for Healthcare Improvement, promotes teamwork through a number of activities. These include a perinatal programme which aims to improve care by applying teamwork interventions such as interprofessional ward rounds and team training opportunities. Another recent development has been the *Patient-centred Medical Home Model* which aims to enhance communication and teamwork, improve coordination of care, expand quality innovations and promote active patient and family involvement (American Academy of Pediatrics, 2009). (For those interested in reading a fuller history of teamwork developments in the US, see Baldwin, 2007.)

Professionals' experiences of teamwork

Having discussed a range of developments in relation to the health and social care professions and their approaches to teamwork, we go on to present a variety of accounts of professionals' *direct experience* of interprofessional teamwork. These vignettes are based on brief semi-structured interviews or email exchanges with colleagues in the field. Specifically, they highlight the range of successes and challenges encountered in different clinical contexts across the world when working in interprofessional teams. We have included them as they provide experiential accounts which help ground and contextualise the more conceptual and theoretical materials we present later in the book.

Successful interprofessional teamwork experiences

Below, nine different professionals reflect upon some of the key successes they have experienced when working in interprofessional teams based in different parts of the world.

In Australia:

In a successful team there's the satisfaction of knowing that the team has performed well even when there have been difficulties associated with the work such as uncontrolled bleeding or a prolonged case. There's also the knowledge that the patient has received the best care possible, and that during the surgery the team worked cohesively together – its 'poetry in motion' to watch. (Nurse, Australia)

As a cardiothoracic surgeon, I am involved in interprofessional teams every day of my working life. In the main, my experiences of teamwork have been very positive. The main successes with interprofessional teamwork have been building up a successful heart and lung transplant/circulatory support service at my previous hospital and at my current institution. Both resulted in excellent patient care and outcomes. (Surgeon, Australia)

In Canada:

With effective teamwork there is a mutual respect for others' contributions. Nursing is seen as important because we spend time with the patient and their family. The rest of the team relies on the nurses for greater understanding. Once the team was familiar that we (nurse practitioners) are not a replacement – they know there is a difference. They can make referrals and there is a real need for nurse practitioners to be involved in patient cases. (Nurse practitioner, Canada)

A holistic approach to health management ensures that the client's assessment and treatment is not subject to splinter areas (e.g. wound care without positioning, bladder retraining without exercise, chemical restraints without trials of alternative measures). Additional successes are sharing of resources, knowledge, product information, sharing of past experience and practises. Efficiency and competency in practice is another by-product of an interprofessional team. Workload sharing and stress reduction is also a significant factor in teamwork. (Occupational therapist, Canada)

In general, my experiences of interprofessional teamwork have been positive. I am part of a family health team. I have always worked closely with nurses. We have now also added a pharmacist, nurse practitioner, dietician and diabetes nurse educator. So the team has grown in last few years. The team is committed to expanding. In fact, the pharmacist has really been a lynch pin. Incorporating her individual and her complementary knowledge has been fantastic. It is mostly due to the team's excitement and openness. (Physician, Canada)

In Norway:

I have had numerous experiences with interprofessional teamwork during 15 years of social work in Norway. Mostly, it has functioned well and improved the client's and their family's situation. Interprofessional teamwork also gives an opportunity to coordinate efforts and have mutual reflections on how to understand the service user's situation which can be very complex. (Social worker, Norway)

In South Africa:

I have had a strong interest in interprofessional teamworking, which developed from my early work in mental health – a clinical area which encouraged teamworking at a much earlier stage than other clinical areas in South Africa. One important early influence was a professor of psychiatry who felt strongly that nurses should be equal partners in caring for people with mental illness. I was encouraged to use and develop my skills and did not ever feel inferior within the team or experience a lack of trust. The culture was that all professionals could contribute but that each was accountable for their actions and would take responsibility for them. (Nurse, South Africa)

In the United Kingdom:

My teamwork successes have included working with mental health service users, their carers and all the professional staff in health and social care. Through listening to all stakeholders and staff, through discussions, assessing, planning, prioritising, checking that resources are available agreement can be reached on the approach to care, support and delivery. This results in teamwork which ensures the delivery of well co-ordinated health and social care services. Working in a team and looking after very disturbed, difficult, aggressive and sometimes violent people, the teamworking approach made the area safe for service users and staff. The service users benefited from a positive environment where they knew who could provide what; and the staff benefited from having a common care approach. (Nurse, UK)

In the United States:

When interprofessional teamwork is successful, patients, families, institutions and professionals benefit. Teamwork is not an intuitive process. It requires education, skills training, ongoing clinical collaboration, and institutional support. It requires time for communication. Professionals need to understand and value the competencies and strengths of each and utilise these competencies to best serve patients. Within each patient situation a different profession may be required to take the lead. Teamwork that functions well allows for leadership to be fluid. It is not always the physician who knows the patient's needs best. However, the professional who best knows the patient may not necessarily know what the patient needs. Teamwork allows for the kind of communication, collaboration and cooperation that sidesteps personalities and works for best patient care. All members must be open to learning from each other and growing in their respective roles. (Social worker, US)

As indicated above, these professionals' reflections on successful teamwork are varied. Highlights of these strengths include coordination of efforts, the need to listen to one another, mutual respect, a commitment to the team, and motivation to learn and share from each other. Importantly, leadership has to be fluid in order to promote effective teamwork and deliver safe, high quality care.

Challenging interprofessional teamwork experiences

In this section, our nine professionals go on to reflect upon some of the key challenges they have encountered when working in different interprofessional teams.

In Australia:

Differences in professional identities give rise to the 'silo' mentality and reduce team cohesion. Although roles within the team are very well-defined, there are times where they overlap and some members may need to compensate or assist more depending on the situation. Additionally, power differentials may stifle communication because lesser experienced members may be reticent to speak up or to ask for clarification when it's necessary. (Nurse, Australia)

The main challenges I have experienced with interprofessional teamwork have been getting all groups on board within the surgical setting. There was initial scepticism about teamwork, but subsequent acceptance emerged. (Surgeon, Australia)

In Canada:

The challenge of effective teamwork is getting existing teams up to speed. It takes time and effort to change the culture. It is really a cultural shift. We have to expose them to teamwork principles. We have to be prepared to move forward. I am not sure that we are good at convincing professionals that it is good to do, or that they are not doing it already. (Nurse practitioner, Canada)

The main challenges on any given team in my experience have been related to personality conflicts, a change in team membership, varying levels of competency or incompetency, absenteeism, inefficient time keeping during meetings and team members who do not think they can learn from others. When the team dynamics change or the team leader becomes more administratively focused and less action orientated, it is a stressor. Health care trends impact on teamwork. Especially with the recent flu outbreak and infection control monitoring in general, these stressors seem to take away from team planning time or meeting time in order to deal with 'acute' situations. (Occupational therapist, Canada)

The biggest challenge right now is integrating the nurse practitioner into our team. We need to figure out what her scope of practice is and then how to integrate it so that it is appropriate for the team. It is important to have that net gain for the team. So, for example, if she is always doing something that needs a consult, then that does not benefit the team. So now it is just figuring out where she fits. It was an easier fit for the dietician and pharmacist who already had a better sense of their scope of practice and how they fit in, but we all are open and work together. (Physician, Canada)

In Norway:

Sometimes interprofessional teamwork has functioned poorly, mostly due to lack of resources. Usually lack of time has been an argument for not giving teamwork the necessary priority. In Norway, interprofessional practice is mandated by the law in our work with children. Perhaps there is an idea that all the professionals will work in a collaborative way, which is not always the case. There is often little support from leaders and the professionals think that interprofessional work is not their responsibility and choose to work more traditionally, which means more individually. I also think we need to focus on interprofessional teamwork during health and social workers' education in order to develop a collaborative attitude. (Social worker, Norway)

In South Africa:

There are number of barriers to teamwork. First, the hierarchical structure of nursing, in which nurses manage themselves at the policy level in opposition to other professional groups. This reinforces professional divides. Nurses at the clinical coalface are influenced in subtle ways by these divides at higher levels. Furthermore, physicians are often brought in as 'experts' to teach nurses, while other professions are not given the same status. In addition, medical training teaches doctors that they can only trust themselves and does not generally encourage them to value the opinions and judgements of other professionals. There's also a sense of 'us' and 'them' – a 'leitmotif' in the South African context which is drawn along multiple lines, including race, gender and profession. (Nurse, South Africa)

In the United Kingdom:

One of the main challenges is dealing with conflict at work – once conflict arises the professionals tend to rush to their profession specific mode. Challenges arise when conflict is related to users, carers and staff. We need to get staff and users to understand that working in a team does not mean giving up their initiatives and decision making to a committee. We need to get staff to work under the leadership which is different from the usual person; getting all the staff to have a common view towards diversity, discrimination, oppression, religion, stigma, gender, ethnicity and race. However it is difficult to get staff to address these challenges. (Nurse, UK)

In the United States:

Interprofessional teamwork is less positive when it is merely a collection of professionals throwing out ideas rather than listening and learning from each other. This happens most often when one member of the 'team' perceives his or her perspective to be most important – when being right surpasses the desire to do what's best for patients. This also seems to occur when a professional or the professional culture does not have an investment in interprofessional work and neither understands nor values input from other disciplines. I've seen patient care jeopardised when teams do not value interprofessional communication. I worked with a paediatric palliative care team that consisted of an oncologist, nurse, social worker, child development specialist, and chaplain. The oncologist and nurse worked together but rarely consulted with the social worker. The social worker had most contact with the children and families but her opinions were not valued. Further, she felt marginalised by the medical professionals. (Social worker, US)

As indicated above, these professionals have outlined a variety of teamwork challenges. Many are underpinned by the power differences that exist in interprofessional teams, which can limit communication and promote friction between members. Other challenges include an uncertainty of how each member 'fits' in the team and pressures on members due to a lack of resources such as time. It was also suggested that limited interprofessional education opportunities may be responsible for why many professionals do not listen to and learn from each other.

Conclusions and implications

Interprofessional teamwork, as we have discussed in this chapter, emerged in a number of countries at different times and in different ways. Despite these differences, it is possible to see that the emergence of teamwork, across these contexts, was related to a common need from policy makers and practitioners – that team-work could help address problems of service delivery which were rooted in poor interprofessional coordination and communication. However, effective teamwork has been found to be a difficult goal to achieve, as it involves a diverse set of requirements, including the need for clear team goals, shared commitment and in-terdependence, ongoing teambuilding efforts, open communication, regular team meetings, as well as mutual respect. The complexities which were described in the teamwork literature were echoed in the professionals' direct accounts of interpro-fessional teamwork, which also included a range of intricate factors related to both their positive and more challenging teamwork experiences. Indeed, it is this com-plexity which underpins teamwork that we go on to examine and discuss, from a number of angles – theoretical, empirical and practical – in the rest of the book.

In this chapter we offered a range of introductory materials to begin to under-stand the width of the different conceptual, political, historical and experiential elements related to interprofessional teamwork. From this starting point, we go in the next chapter to explore how teamwork has moved to occupy a central posi-tion within many health and social care systems as a key approach to enhance the delivery of care.

2 Current developments affecting interprofessional teamwork

Introduction

As we noted in the previous chapter, there have been numerous arguments as well as policy documents from national governments, professional regulatory bodies and international agencies which have repeatedly demanded that health and social care professions work in a more collaborative, team-based manner. From these materials, it is possible to identify a range of developments which have emerged as current 'drivers' for the promotion of interprofessional teamwork. We review these developments to explore how they have contributed to promoting teamwork across the globe. While we have attempted to provide a comprehensive account of current teamwork developments, this chapter is more indicative than definitive in nature. In this chapter we also present the views of five teamwork leaders who discuss the current gaps in our knowledge of interprofessional teamwork. Collectively, these leaders' views offer an insight into what is currently 'missing' in relation to our understanding of teamwork – content which we aim to address in the later sections of the book. Finally, we outline a range of conclusions and implications for interprofessional teamwork.

Quality and safety

Improving the quality and safety of care has, in recent years, been a key driver for the use of interprofessional teamwork, as the need for effective collaboration and communication is seen as central for achieving such gains. Arguably, the focus on delivering a quality service is linked with the rise of many of the other developments, such as the patient-centred movement and consumerisation (see below) as well as the emergence of a number of quality improvement initiatives (see Chapter 3). Encouragingly, a small number of studies have indicated that interprofessional teamwork can contribute to improved quality in the following areas: reducing patient complaints, increasing patient satisfaction, and reducing stress and burnout among professions (e.g. Beckman *et al.*, 1994; Wofford *et al.*, 2004). However, at present, the rigour and quantity of this research are still rather limited.

In relation to safety, concerns can be traced back to Ivan Illich's (1977) seminal book entitled *Limits to Medicine* in which he argued that the medicalisation of society caused more harm than good; and often rendered many people, in effect, life-long patients. Through the use of a range of health statistics, Illich demonstrated the extent of post-operative side effects and drug-induced illness, which he termed *iatrogenic* – physician-induced – disease.

The publication in 2000 of the Institute of Medicine's (IoM) report, *To Err is Human*, re-ignited both public and professional interest in safety and the reduction of errors (Kohn *et al.*, 2000). Based on data from US medical record studies dating back to 1984, it was found that there were between 44 000 and 98 000 adverse events reported each year. The IoM report went on to state that in order to identify error, each team member needed to know their own responsibilities, as well as those of their members. Recommendations to prevent error included that health and social care organisations should begin to implement patient-safety programmes that trained professionals to work effectively together in teams.

Since the publication of this report, a range of patient-safety initiatives (e.g. checklists) have been developed to improve the quality of team communication and interprofessional relations (e.g. Awad *et al.*, 2005; Haynes *et al.*, 2009) (also see Chapter 6). In addition, a number of organisations promoting interprofessional teamwork and patient safety have been established such as the UK National Patient Safety Agency, the US Institute for Healthcare Improvement, the Australian Patient Safety Foundation and the World Health Organization's World Alliance for Patient Safety. A range of interprofessional patient-safety initiatives has also emerged from these organisations. For example, the Canadian Patient Safety Institute (2008) recently published its interprofessional competencies aimed at enhancing collaborative knowledge, skills and behaviours related to safety.

Despite improvements in quality and safety, Wachter (2004) has argued that error-reporting systems have had little impact, and scant progress had been made in improving professionals' accountability. Indeed, a recent national survey of medical residents' perceptions of intra- and interprofessional conflict and error undertaken by Baldwin and Daugherty (2008) found that of the 523 residents who reported conflict with at least one other professional, 36% reported that it was linked to a 'serious medical error'. Of the 187 reporting conflict with two or more other professionals, the serious medical error rate was 51%. A recent qualitative study provides further information on how professionals perceive error (Box 2.1), and suggests that a better understanding of these perceptions may be helpful in designing systems to improve patient safety.

Patient-centred care

According to Jewson (1976) in his paper on the 'disappearance of the sick man', care in the 1700s was patient-centred. Physicians, he argued, at that time were very responsive to the needs of their usually rich patrons. However, towards the end of that century, this relationship altered. The production of medical knowledge was assumed by medical investigators. This changed the practice of medicine from

> **Box 2.1** Operating room team members' perceptions of error.
>
> Espin *et al.* (2006) explored perceptions of errors in the context of team-based surgical care. Their study provided a rare qualitative insight into the common justifications used by professionals to explain why they perceive some and not other events as 'errors'. The authors found that surgeons, anaesthesiologists and nurses were remarkably consistent in terms of error identification. In particular, physicians and nurses tended to define error primarily as deviation from standards of practice. Events not addressed in current standards, and which did not result in clear harm to the patient, were often regarded, fatalistically, as 'acts of God'.

being negotiated between physician and patient to a consensus of opinion imposed from the growing community of publicly funded medical researchers.

The modern notion of 'patient-centred care' was introduced into the health literature in the mid-1950s by Balint (1955, 1956), who compared it to 'illness-centred medicine' (Brown, 1999). The concept emerged from the paradigm of holism, which suggests that people need to be seen in their bio-psychosocial entirety (Henbest and Stewart, 1989), and focuses the attention of health care providers on patients' individual identities (Armstrong, 1982; Lewin *et al.*, 2001; Beach *et al.*, 2006). The main features of patient-centredness include health and social care providers sharing control of consultations, decisions about interventions or the management of the health problems with their patients, and a focus in consultations on the patient as a person, rather than solely on the disease (Lewin *et al.*, 2001). This may involve shared decision-making to develop a treatment plan, listening to patients' experience of illness and forming a patient–doctor relationship based on empathy and care.

There is a growing literature arguing for the adoption of patient-centred care in the delivery of health and social care services (e.g. Stewart, 1995; Amey *et al.*, 2006). The inclusion of the patient in the care process is viewed as important for it allows professionals to tailor their care to respond to the different needs of different individuals. As the UK Nursing and Midwifery Council (2002, section 4.2) stated, 'patients and clients are equal partners in their care and therefore have the right to be involved in the health care team's decisions'.

More recently, the notion of patient-centred care has come to embrace a collaborative, team-based approach. The focus has expanded to include all health and social care professionals working together, with the patients at the centre, to improve the quality of the services they deliver (e.g. Dean, 2008).

As Herbert (2005, p. 2) has noted:

Collaborative patient-centred practice is designed to promote the active participation of each discipline in patient care. It enhances patient- and family-centred goals and values, provides mechanisms for continuous communication among care givers, optimises staff participation in clinical decision making within and across disciplines, and fosters respect for disciplinary contributions of all professionals.

Box 2.2 The development of collaborative patient-centred practice in Canada.

The key drivers for collaborative patient-centred practice can be traced back to Roy Romanow's (2002) report, entitled *Building on values: The Future of Health Care in Canada*, in which he stressed that the future of health care needed 'providers ... to work together and share expertise in a team environment' (p. 109). This in turn would ensure that care would be 'shaped around the needs of individual patients, their families and communities' (p. 50). The *First Ministers' Accord* (Health Canada, 2003) echoed Romanow's sentiments about collaborative and patient-centred care. To help implement the recommendations in both reports, Health Canada launched its IECPCP (*Interprofessional Education for Collaborative Patient-Centred Practice*) initiative, which funded 20 projects across Canada to plan, develop and deliver a range of interprofessional activities across acute and community settings (Health Canada, 2009).

Box 2.2 offers an example of how in Canada the adoption of collaborative patient-centred practice has been significant in the past few years.

By including patients as part of the team, this approach assumes they can be given the opportunity to increase their knowledge of care. It also provides opportunities for professionals to increase their knowledge of the patient and their individual health and social care needs. In addition, it has been argued that a patient-centred team approach could act as a method of disease prevention (Dean, 2008) and may also allow the patient to recover in a positive environment (Edwards, 2002).

While efforts to advance patient-centred team practice are laudable, there are a number of challenges. For example, in order for patients and their families to play a successful role in an interprofessional team, it is important that both they and their care providers learn how to work within these contexts. Such learning creates an extra burden for both patients and professionals. Also, one needs to be mindful that imbalances of power exist between patients and professionals – traditionally professionals have controlled health and social care interactions. Indeed, there is little evidence to suggest that any systemic transfer of control from professional to patient has in effect occurred.

Shift towards chronic conditions

In the past 25 years we have experienced a shift from acute to chronic illnesses such as arthritis, hypertension and diabetes. This is linked to shifting demographics – people are living longer, and the burden of complex chronic conditions which occur in later life has grown accordingly (Strong *et al.*, 2005; World Health Organization, 2005). For example, in the UK it has been reported that chronic illness affects six in ten adults, but this burden of illness is particularly severe among older people, affecting two-thirds of those aged over 75 – nearly three million people (Office for National Statistics, 2002). In North America it is estimated that the percentage of people aged 65 years and older will double from the current 13% to approximately 25% in the next 20 years (Medical Advisory Secretariat, 2008). Many low- and middle-income countries face a similar situation. By 2030, for instance, it is anticipated that China's population of people over the age of 65 years will increase from 7 to 16% (National Bureau of Statistics of China, 2009).

The growth of disease from chronic conditions has meant that the acute care models on which most health systems have been based since World War II are no longer seen as the most appropriate way of delivering services. Health and social care professionals, it has been suggested, need to work together to ensure that they can respond to and manage these chronic (and often complex and long-term) illnesses (World Health Organization, 2005). However, this rise in chronic illness does not necessarily mean that policies recommending more interprofessional teamwork and greater integration of services will be implemented. For example, Cott et al. (2008) undertook a qualitative study which explored the relevance of traditional chronic care uniprofessional models in comparison with interprofessional models, and found no evidence for the widespread use of formal collaborative interprofessional teamwork. Typically, professions working in this context preferred traditional uniprofessional models of care delivery.

Media coverage of teamworking

The media – television, radio, newspapers and the internet – are extremely powerful tools in shaping the way that people perceive the world. The media's role in affecting health and social care policy and in changing the public's perceptions of care has been regarded as critical (Otten, 1992; Seale, 2003, 2004). Today, the media often provides reports of adverse care due to poor interprofessional teamwork and collaboration. Recent instances of the media reporting such examples include problematic care delivered to cancer patients in the Netherlands, where limited coordination and communication were reported among oncology teams (Dutch News, 2009); and poor interprofessional interactions between nurses and physicians in the US, where a nurse described being belittled by a physician after paging him during the night for a seemingly non-urgent case (Terkin, 2008).

Well-publicised failures of interprofessional collaboration have been at the centre of many health and social care inquiries over the past 25 years, such as the Cleveland child abuse inquiry (Butler-Sloss, 1988) and the Victoria Climbié inquiry (Laming, 2003) in the UK. Furthermore, Kennedy's (2001) report on the death of babies undergoing heart surgery, also in the UK, found that while surgeons considered themselves as effective team players, this contrasted with the perceptions of their colleagues, from other professions, who saw their approach to teamwork in more problematic terms. Similarly, the Justice St Claire report in Canada found that in the cases of the multiple sentinel events and incidents at the children's hospital cardiac operating room (OR), nurses reported concerns about a surgeon's practice were largely ignored as they were perceived as not capable judges of surgical performance (Sinclair, 2000). Indeed, OR nurses' comments on surgeons' practice were deemed to be inappropriate as they were outside their scope of practice. Such extreme cases may be rare, and usually linked to systemic failures in which poor interprofessional teamwork contributed in part to the problem, not its entirety.

Rising consumerism within health care

Today patients are (or have the potential to be) more informed about the nature of their health conditions and their care than previously. They and their families can access a wide range of sources – the media, patient organisations, pressure groups and professional organisations – which can provide them with insights into the nature of their illness and their health and care services. Access to a wide range of health care information through the internet (through both specialised care sites and more general information sites such as Wikipedia) has further contributed to the growth in patient awareness of health and social care issues, although the quality of this information is very variable (Eysenbach *et al.*, 2002). Patients are also increasingly encouraged to participate in care through government initiatives such as expert patient programmes (e.g. UK Expert Patients Programme, 2009).

Increasing patient awareness, empowerment and responsibility can be linked to the notion of *consumerism* in health and social care, as several authors have discussed in relation to the growing centrality of consumerism and patient choice within UK health policies (Newman and Vidler, 2006; Greener, 2009). Changing relationships between consumers and providers may have impacts on interprofessional teamworking. For example, consumers and their carers are being drawn increasingly together in different care teams through programmes such as lay self-management and policy initiatives such as collaborative patient-centred practice (see Box 2.2).

While such developments have appeared to shift attention towards the patient and their family, one needs to consider the actual nature of a patients' role within health and social care teams. As we noted above, the balance of power between patients and professionals has traditionally favoured the latter. It is still unclear how consumerism may have affected these historical imbalances. Arguably, professionals still hold the dominant position in managing care due to their control of, or central role in, many aspects of this process.

Rising costs of care

Every year the cost of providing health and social care services rises. In some years, expenditure rises slowly, in others, for example, the past decade or so, more rapidly (Ginsburg, 2004). These budgetary increases in cost of care have been an important element in various governments' interest in interprofessional teamwork. Reorganising services to provide a more coordinated, collaborative, team-oriented approach has been seen as a way of reducing duplication, improving efficiency and effectiveness as well as helping to contain costs (Ingram and Desombre, 1999; McPherson *et al.*, 2001).

Pressures from governments to decrease patient lengths of stay as a way to contain rises in the cost of care within acute inpatient institutions are widespread (e.g. Rice, 1992; Ikegami and Campbell, 2004; Bodenheimer, 2005). With such decreases in inpatient length of stay, the need for effective interprofessional teamwork becomes more pressing. Communication between professionals becomes increasingly important; as patients enter and exit the inpatient care setting more quickly and professionals have less time to communicate with one another. Advances in information technology or IT (see below) have the capacity to help with communication especially when more than one team is involved in patient care. For example, electronic medical record systems allow each team member to have quick access to up-to-date patient information and are being implemented rapidly into health systems in a range of settings, although evidence regarding efficiency gains remains weak (Poissant et al., 2005).

While some studies have indicated that interprofessional teamwork can help reduce costs (e.g. Zwarenstein et al., 2009), the quality and quantity of this evidence are still rather limited. For example, at the time of writing we could not find a review on cost-effectiveness of using interprofessional teamwork to deliver care. As we go on to note (see Chapter 7), a good deal of the evidence on teamwork rests upon members' perceptions of their own collaborative performances.

A focus on rural care

Often overshadowed by the complexities of urban care, the needs of rural communities have increasingly come in focus in the past decade (e.g. Australian Institute of Health and Welfare, 2008). This focus is timely given that, for instance, the US Department of Health and Human Services (2003) has estimated that 20 million of a potential 70 million rural Americans have inadequate access to health care. In addition, as the Institute of Medicine (2004a) points out, rural communities represent nearly 20% of the US population and, like urban counterparts, they are rich in cultural diversity. However, delivering care in rural communities, in high, low- and middle-income country settings, presents a number of challenges. Providing coordinated care to large geographically remote areas is particularly difficult, as is recruiting and retaining health and social professionals to work in these regions (Chopra et al., 2008; Grobler et al., 2009).

Interprofessional teamwork in rural communities also faces a number of challenges. Typically, team members need to work across large areas which means opportunities for interactions are restricted. In addition, shortages of professionals based in these regions may mean that they need to work outside of their own professional boundaries to deliver the services of their colleagues who may only visit periodically (Blue and Fitzgerald, 2002). In addition, due to the absence of physicians in many rural settings, physician assistants and nurse practitioners often have an expanded role in providing care (Hooker and McCaig, 2001). While this helps to ensure better access to care, possible tensions with professional role overlap have been reported (e.g. Booth and Hewison, 2002). These elements are examined in more depth in Chapters 4 and 5.

Professional associations

A professional association (sometimes called a professional body or society) is an organisation whose aim is to further the interests of its members. Professional associations such as the UK Royal College of Nursing, the Danish Medical Association and the American Physical Therapy Association are involved in the development and monitoring of professional education programmes, updating skills, regulating entry and maintaining professional standards. They are therefore central in the certification process which allows individual professionals to practice.

As previously noted, professional associations representing the spectrum of the health and social care professions have been calling increasingly for their members to be prepared to work effectively in interprofessional teams. For example, in the UK, the Nursing and Midwifery Council (2002) stated in its *Code of Professional Conduct* that qualified nurses and midwives:

> Are expected to work co-operatively within teams and to respect the skills, expertise and contributions of your colleagues. (section 4.2)

Similar statements can be found in the documents of professional regulatory bodies for other professions, such as physicians (General Medical Council, 2001), occupational therapists (College of Occupational Therapists, 2000) and social workers (International Federation of Social Workers, 2009). In the US, for example, the Accreditation Council for Graduate Medical Education (ACGME) revised the lists of competencies for physicians to include aspects of interprofessional coordination and collaboration (ACGME, 2007).

While professional regulatory bodies have a central role in promoting teamwork in their published documentation, it is unclear how effectively their policy statements are being implemented. As we discuss later in the book, these associations play a role in protecting and advancing their members' social, economic and political interests. As a result, there seems to be a contradiction in their demands for interprofessional teamwork, on the one hand, and the representation of their members' profession-specific interests, on the other.

Teamwork funding

Another key driver for the growth of interprofessional teamwork has been the funding provided nationally and regionally by governments across the globe to design, implement and evaluate a range of different interprofessional team-based programmes, courses, initiatives and interventions. In the UK, for example, in the past few years the Department of Health has funded a number of team-based initiatives (see Box 2.3).

Also, as noted in Box 2.2 (see above), Health Canada has provided substantial funding, through its *Interprofessional Education for Collaborative Patient-Centred Practice* initiative, to establish a wide variety of interprofessional initiatives across the country. In other settings, including Australia, Brazil and South Africa, both public

Box 2.3   A recently funded study on interprofessional teamwork in stroke care.

Funded by the National Institute of Health Research Service Delivery and Organisation programme (NIHR SDO), the 'Interprofessional teamwork across stroke care pathways: outcome and patient and carer experience' study is based at Kingston University and St. George's, University of London, UK. The study was commissioned to explore the interaction between the contexts and mechanisms of interprofessional teamwork that influence patients' and carers' experience of care and clinical outcomes. It uses mixed methods and has five phases:

1. Organisational and service delivery contexts are being mapped within the acute and primary and social care sectors. Interviews with key staff are also being undertaken to explore organisational structures, care pathways, governance and mechanisms for teamwork.
2. Anonymised patient data are being retrieved from the hospital stroke registers at three and twelve months for functional independence, anxiety and depression, mortality, recurrence and reintegration to normal living. In this phase stroke teams are completing a survey to assess team function.
3. A sub-sample of patients and family carers are being recruited and interviewed about their experience of stroke care. These interviews are being repeated on two further occasions: during rehabilitation and on their return home.
4. Interviews with professionals working in hospital and community stroke teams about their experience of teamwork are being conducted and selected observations of team meetings are being undertaken.
5. Data across the phases are being analysed to interrogate associations between the nature of teamwork with the severity of stroke, the progress of rehabilitation and the quality of the patient and carer experience. Preliminary analyses are being fed back to participating teams with the aim of promoting better understanding of how interprofessional teamwork influences stroke outcomes.

Two advisory groups support the study: a service user and carer advisory group to ensure the study is grounded in the perspective of the service user and their carers; and also a professional advisory group. The report will be available by late 2011 at www.sdo.nihr.ac.uk/.

and private funding sources have also supported the development of interprofessional teamwork.

Championing teamwork

The past decade has witnessed a growth in the number of organisations which have been established to promote interprofessional teamwork, collaboration and education. For example, over the past 20 years the Centre for the Advancement of Interprofessional Education (CAIPE) has actively promoted a range of interprofessional initiatives within the UK. Similarly, the Canadian Interprofessional Health Collaborative (CIHC) which was formed in 2006 has begun to coordinate efforts within Canada to promote interprofessional education, collaboration and teamwork between health and social care organisations, health educators, students, researchers and professionals. A similar initiative was recently started in the US in the form of the American Interprofessional Health Collaborative (AIHC). While it has a broader mandate, the Institute for Healthcare Improvement has been helping to lead the interprofessional activities within the context of improving the quality of health care in the US. The Australasian Interprofessional Practice and Education Network (AIPPEN) was also recently formed to help coordinate information exchange, communication and partnership for a range of interprofessional activities across Australia and New Zealand.

Appendix 5 provides further information and web links for these and other organisations which promote a range of interprofessional activities.

Through their work – reports, conferences and resources – these organisations have helped enhance understanding of a range of interprofessional activities. They have also championed the interprofessional agenda by liaising with, and lobbying, policy makers, practitioners, students and patients. However, as we discuss later, not all of these initiatives have been underpinned by robust evidence of the effectiveness in improving teamwork, patient satisfaction and outcomes.

Information technology

There has been an expansion in the use of IT for both work and leisure purposes as economies of scale make IT much more affordable. The expansion has led to the development of several forms of electronic communication with the potential for improving interprofessional teamwork and collaboration.

Traditionally, teamwork has been an activity which was undertaken in the same space, largely through synchronous interaction. However, the development of accessible and reliable IT offers opportunities to engage in newer forms of teamwork. Increasingly, IT such as the internet, video and computer conferencing are being employed as they offer possibilities to enhance interprofessional interaction across space and time.

As Reeves and Freeth (2003, p. 81) point out:

These technologies can offer an *electronic bridge* to ensure that practitioners can communicate either synchronously or asynchronously.

Furthermore, it has been argued that the increasing use of these different forms of IT will alter the nature of interprofessional teamwork. As the Registered Nurses Association of Ontario (2006, p. 19) has stated:

The composition, context and structure of teams is also changing to include virtual teams, that provide care using video and telecommunications technology without ever meeting in person.

Indeed, it has been argued that the use of IT will affect future interprofessional interactions (e.g. Careau *et al.*, 2008). Professions who traditionally dominated face-to-face team interactions will be no more visible than their colleagues who would say little in such conventional interactions. These professionals can now potentially interact in a much more significant manner by the use of electronic communication. However, as a number of authors have found, the use of varying types of communication technologies can also be interruptive for practitioners (Coiera and Toombs, 1998; Hartswood *et al.*, 2003). Box 2.4 outlines other challenges which can emerge for team members when new IT systems are implemented.

Box 2.4   IT and teamwork.

Scott *et al.* (2005) examined primary care team members' perceptions of the implementation of an electronic medical record system in a non-profit health care organisation in the US. Qualitative interviews were undertaken with clinicians and managers based in four primary care teams. Findings indicated that the initial decision to introduce the system was seen as remote from team members. Many members felt the system was not effective for the local environment, sparking doubt and resistance. Problems with software development increased local resistance, as clinicians' productivity and ability to collaborate decreased. The authors go on to conclude that the implementation of new IT systems needs much more careful attention to team members' needs as well as meeting the demands of the local environment.

The security of electronic patient information is a further concern (for example, see Mannan *et al.*, 2006; Anderson, 2008). Confidential information needs to be protected from hackers who may infiltrate systems as well as from accidental security breaches or loss. However, robust data security systems may make the use of electronic information portals more cumbersome and time-consuming for professionals, undermining some of the advantages of such systems. In addition, ongoing training is required to ensure that team members can use the technology effectively in their interactions.

Evolution of professional work

Advances in scientific knowledge, coupled with the ability to use more complex technologies and procedures, have led to the evolution of professional work and greater specialisation in health and social care. For example, it has been suggested that dealing with patients' often complex needs, such as within palliative care, requires a team of specialised health and social care professionals (e.g. Cadell *et al.*, 2007). In addition, new medical specialities, such as neonatology; new specialist roles, such as advance practice nurses; and new supporting roles, such as physician assistants, have emerged. This wide range of providers need to work collaboratively, often in interprofessional teams, to provide patient care. However, while greater specialisation may be needed to manage and deliver more complex interventions and technologies, it can also lead to larger divisions between and within professions. These, in turn, may influence the relations between professions as well as between organisations of different professionals. Greater specialisation may lead to the increasing fragmentation of care, as more and varying types of practitioners are involved in delivering care in different ways, at different points and in different organisations in the care trajectory. As we discuss later, teamwork can therefore be a difficult goal to achieve regularly and routinely, despite being a key goal for health and social services.

This situation may be compounded by the growing participation of lay providers, as well as by other developments such as the greater involvement of patients and carers in health care decision-making (see above). These elements may add further complexity to the delivery of care. This contemporary picture of health and social care contrasts quite starkly with the traditional 'profession-centric' manner in which care was often provided in the past – without any input from the lay community.

A further more recent development in the evolution of professional work in Canada, Europe and the US has been the introduction of new working regulations which limit the hours that can be worked by junior physicians and other groups. These new regulations have renewed the focus on how teamwork can compensate for the shorter shifts, and therefore the increased number of staff involved in care that need to accommodate these restrictions.

As professional roles continue to shift and evolve, new challenges for teamworking are likely to emerge and novel ways of promoting interaction will need to be developed and evaluated.

Education and training

To help ensure effective interprofessional team performance, it has been argued that individuals need a range of collaborative attributes: attitudes, knowledge and skills (Barr *et al.*, 2005; Reeves *et al.*, 2008). For instance, team members require a comprehensive understanding of their own professional roles and those of their colleagues. Teamwork also requires the skills to work as an effective team member and attitudes that underpin a collaborative approach. It is commonly argued, however, that professionals tend to lack these attributes as traditionally teamwork has not been included in their pre- or post-qualification training (e.g. Barr *et al.*, 2005; Reeves, 2008). Indeed, this traditional absence of learning how to collaborate appears, in some way, to be based upon an assumption that professionals will *intuitively* know how to work collaboratively. Although, as we have noted above, evidence related to continued failures in communication and collaboration across health care systems remind us that this is not the case. Also, as we have outlined above, due to demographic and health system changes, there is a *pressing* need for professionals to be able to collaborate in an effective interprofessional manner.

As a result, health and social care education providers have been increasingly offering pre- and post-qualification programmes, modules and workshops which provide students and practising professionals with a range of learning activities aimed to help them understand the principles of collaboration in order to perform effectively as an interprofessional team player (e.g. Barr *et al.*, 2005). At the same time, a number of professional regulatory bodies have stressed the need for educational providers to design and deliver a range of interprofessional learning experiences (e.g. General Medical Council, 2001; Nursing and Midwifery Council, 2002). Moreover, there has been a growth in the development of 'benchmark statements' and competency frameworks to ensure that learners develop the appropriate knowledge attitudes and skills of teamwork (e.g. Barr, 1998; Verma *et al.*, 2006; Quality Assurance Agency for Higher Education, 2009). Indeed, the use of these approaches has stimulated discussion on how teamwork and collaboration attributes can be appropriately assessed and measured. Although, as one of us recently argued, the use of competency-based approaches can be problematic as they can fail to capture the essence of working in an interprofessional manner (Reeves *et al.*, 2009a). There can also be other difficulties linked to the use of interprofessional competencies. The Royal College of Physicians and Surgeons of Canada (2005) competency framework, for example, requires physicians to develop competences to collaborate as team members as well as competencies to be the leaders of interprofessional teams – a tension which we explore later in the book.

Some current gaps in our understanding of teamwork

Having outlined a range of important developments which have promoted interprofessional teamwork, in this part of the chapter we offer the views from five interprofessional leaders on current *gaps* in our knowledge of teamwork. These extracts are based on short semi-structured interviews with each of these leaders. They help to highlight some key areas in which there is only a limited understanding of teamwork.

A view from Canada:

We need to understand that we do not educate people to work in interprofessional teams and that they go out into the healthcare system thinking that they are working in teams.

They need to be educated on certain factors such as barriers like where stereotypes come from, how gender affects teams and use of language. The problem is that we do not educate and train in post secondary institutions. We assume that students can do it – this is a bad assumption. Also, the health care industry has not understood that they are not only a service organization, they are a learning system as well. Very little attention has been paid to develop the learning side of the health care system. (Teamwork leader 1, Canada)

There are a number of gaps between perceptions that interprofessional practice is what health professionals are already doing. Hence leading to knowledge gaps in what collaborative team practice is all about; in health professionals realising the value of having patients and their families as part of the team; in the rhetoric around patient centred care and the actual realisation of the same; in knowing what constitutes collaborative practice; in knowing how to and then executing effective teamwork among health professionals; in knowing what the roles, knowledge and skills are between different health disciplines. (Teamwork leader 2, Canada)

A view from the UK:

Staff from the different professions working in health and social care often recognise that they must work together. However, because they have not had any education and training in teamworking, they are unable to realise its benefits. They work together but the subtleties, the mechanisms and the understanding of interprofessional working in a team is not always present in their thinking. Furthermore, power struggles, ideological and theoretical differences add to the challenges for the team. (Teamwork leader 3, UK)

A view from the US:

I think there is beginning to be a plethora of competency frameworks for teamwork training from different perspectives that is going to need to be sorted out. I also think that to truly transform education and teamwork training for practitioners in the clinical setting we need to move backward from competency preparation to focus on fundamental values and knowledge about each other to reshape professional identities. I also think that teamwork and collaboration are relational processes that apply in many, many circumstances of care delivery. However, our current preoccupation with 'teams' blocks our vision to the larger agenda of collaborative processes that take many forms – collaborative decision-making, care coordination, problem solving 'huddles' in a micro-system, at the organization level, and in larger professional and political contexts. (Teamwork leader 4, US)

I think that the biggest two gaps are related – theory and research. We need to develop and refine theories and theoretical frameworks that guide the development of collaboration and teamwork. The development of theory can also help inform research and evaluation efforts. Theories can help predict what we think should happen with interventions, and then we need research and evaluation to determine whether they have happened. The areas of greatest need for research, I believe, relate to measuring the effectiveness of interventions in achieving the development of teamwork knowledge and skills in students, and then assessing whether these are used and maintained in the practice setting. Clinically or with respect to practice, we need more and better-designed research to gauge the impact of team care on patient outcomes and the costs of care. (Teamwork leader 5, US)

The leaders' views coalesce around two main issues: a need to further develop the theoretical and empirical knowledge of teamwork; and a need to focus on the design, implementation and evaluation of interventions that effectively promote teamwork. In subsequent chapters we explore these issues in more depth in an effort to understand them and provide ideas for addressing them. We return to these leaders in Chapter 9 when they provide their ideas about the future for interprofessional teamwork.

Conclusions and implications

As we have outlined above, the need for interprofessional teamwork can be identified in a number of different political, social, economic, organisational, educational and professional developments which have emerged in the past decade or so. Collectively, these developments have given more attention to a need for health and social care professions to work together in the delivery of care. While these developments have helped place interprofessional teamwork at the forefront of approaches to resolve service delivery problems, as the interprofessional leaders have pointed out, there remain a number of theoretical and empirical gaps in our understanding of interprofessional teamwork.

3 Interprofessional teamwork: key concepts and issues

Introduction

The previous two chapters helped to set the scene for the book by mapping the emergence of teamwork and describing a range of current developments. In this chapter we aim to explore key concepts and issues related to interprofessional teamwork to understand its conceptual foundations. In doing so, we review and critique the literature describing teamwork characteristics, team typologies and the constituent elements that contribute to team effectiveness. We also argue for a *contingency* approach to teamwork – one which values other forms of interprofessional work such as collaboration, coordination and networking. Finally, we explore the applicability of teamwork approaches that have been developed in other settings (e.g. crew resource management) for health and social care settings.

Describing and characterising teamwork

Interprofessional teams come into existence to ensure that health and social care professions can complete a care task (or combination of tasks) that they could not achieve so effectively on their own. Indeed, as we outlined in Chapter 1, the increasing complexity of organising, coordinating and delivering care demands that professionals regularly come together, share information and reach agreement in their work. However, as we go on to discuss, not all groups of practitioners who come together to collaborate work as teams.

Traditionally, the literature has employed terms such as 'group' and 'team' interchangeably (e.g. Douglas, 1983; Adair, 1986). The rationale behind this standpoint is that interactions which occur within groups and teams are similar. As Douglas (1983, p. 1) noted:

> Teams are co-operative groups in that they are called into being to perform a task, a task that cannot be performed by an individual.

More recently, authors have moved away from thinking that groups and teams are interchangeable concepts. While the former is seen as a 'looser' arrangement of individuals who periodically interact, the latter is regarded as something more. Sundstrom *et al.* (1990), for instance, have emphasised three core elements that characterise teams. First, individuals should hold a shared identity of themselves as 'team members'. Second, each team member should have their own individual role so as to ensure that members do not duplicate work. Third, teams should share a collective agreement around how they work together.

Similarly, Pritchard (1995) has outlined four distinctive features that help define a team. While one feature – that team members should have an understanding of all members' role and function – is similar to one of the elements proposed by Sundstrom *et al.*, Pritchard also identifies a number of additional features: team members should share a common purpose for their work; members pool their skills and knowledge; and team members are able to work interdependently with one another.

Mohrman *et al.*'s (1995) description shares a number of similar elements, including that team members share goals; are interdependent in their accomplishment of tasks and goals; and that they work in an integrated fashion with one another. In addition, they emphasise that a team needs to be mutually and collectively accountable for meeting goals and producing outputs. Cohen and Bailey (1997) outline similar features, but importantly also note that teams are regarded (by their members and others) as discrete social entities.

In their approach, Headrick *et al.* (1998) suggest a range of characteristics which describe interprofessional teamwork. These include that team goals and objectives are stated, restated and reinforced; that member roles and tasks are clear and known; that the atmosphere in the team is respectful; that responsibility for team success is shared; that there is clarity regarding authority and accountability; that the team decision-making and communication processes are clear; and that information is regularly shared.

Teamwork characteristics put forward by these authors overlap substantially. Table 3.1 summarises and synthesises these descriptions of teams to identify key elements which comprise the essence of teamwork.

As illustrated in Table 3.1, our synthesis produced over 20 descriptors of teamwork. From this starting point we have identified five common elements of teamwork: shared identity, clear roles/tasks/goals, interdependence of team members, integration of work and shared responsibility.

Team tasks

While these five elements help define the essence of a team, for us, they overlook *team tasks* and how, in particular their predictability, urgency and complexity can affect teamwork. In clinical settings such as operating theatres, intensive care and trauma care where team tasks are typically unpredictable, urgent and complex professionals need to have a close interdependence, integration and shared responsibility. In contrast, in settings such as primary care or outpatient clinics, where team tasks are generally more predictable and less urgent, issues such as interdependence and integration of members' may be equally important, but less

Table 3.1 Synthesising some elements of teamwork.

Author	Description	Shared elements
Sundstrom *et al.*	Shared team identity Clear individual roles Collective work agreement	
Mohrman *et al.*	Work together Mutual accountability Shared goals Team interdependence Team integration	
Pritchard	Common purpose Understanding of roles/functions Pooled skills/knowledge Team independence	Shared team identity Clear roles/tasks/goals → Interdependence Integration Shared responsibility
Cohen and Bailey	Interdependent tasks Shared responsibility Shared team identity	
Headrick *et al.*	Clear team goals/objectives Clear roles/tasks Respectful team atmosphere Shared responsibility Clarity regarding authority/accountability Clear team decision-making processes Open communication/information sharing	

urgent, and are thus generally organised in a less structured fashion. Box 3.1 provides two examples – the operating room and the outpatient clinic – of how predictability, urgency and complexity can have an influence on the ability of interprofessional teams to function.

Box 3.1   The influence of team tasks on teamwork.

The operating room. Time pressures and divergent workflow patterns within this context can minimise opportunities for teamwork, necessitating tight prior planning for interprofessional collaboration and placing a high demand on clarity of roles and team communication. Work in the operating room involves critical sources of variability. The patient's arrival can be emergent and not scheduled. Further, the surgical process, the patient condition and results of the intervention can be unpredictable.

The arthritis outpatient clinic. Patients and their families arrive at the clinic at scheduled times. During the appointment there can be a discussion between patient, family and different professionals about their arthritis care. Either at or after the appointment, an interprofessional review of treatment may take place during which plans for the future, which may include referral to other services and a date for a return visit. A consistent group of professionals may share care, often asynchronously.

As Box 3.1 indicates, due to the unpredictable, urgent and complex nature of work in the operating room, there is a clear need for an effective time-critical inter-professional team response, which contrasts with more predictable and routinised nature of the outpatient clinic. We return, later in this chapter, to explore how team tasks relate to the shared elements outlined in Table 3.1.

Team typologies

Teamwork authors have also provided a range of different typologies for varying types of teams. In general, these suggest that teams can be placed on a spectrum from 'poor teams' (e.g. those who do not work in an integrated fashion and interact infrequently) to 'good teams' (those who share an integrated approach and inter-act on a regular basis). Below we summarise a number of the more well-known typologies before offering a critique.

Bruce (1980) devised a model of teamwork that includes three types of teams. The first type is a *nominal* team in which members do not share a common goal; may have little idea of each other's roles; where communication is poor; and where there is generally little interaction between members. The second is a *convenient* team in which a few members share a common goal; there is some understanding of members' roles and responsibilities; but where there is only limited interaction and communication between members. The third is a *committed* team in which all members share a common goal; roles and responsibilities between team members are well understood; and where there is good communication and regular interac-tion between members.

Katzenbach and Smith (1993) developed a slightly different model that contains five types of team:

- *Working groups* in which members hold some shared information and under-take some team activities, but where there is no joint responsibility or clear definition of team roles
- *Pseudo teams* in which members are labelled as a 'team' but, in reality, have little shared responsibility or coordination of their teamwork
- *Potential teams* in which members are beginning to work in a collaborative man-ner but have few of the factors needed for effective teamwork, such as the shar-ing of common team goals
- *Real teams* in which members share common goals and share some accountabil-ity
- *High performance teams* in which members all hold a clear understanding of their roles, all share common team goals and, in addition, encourage members' per-sonal development.

More recently, Drinka and Clark (2000) have distinguished between the follow-ing types of multidisciplinary or interdisciplinary health care teams. The first is an *ad hoc task group* who work together to solve task-related problems and then disbands. The second is a *formal multidisciplinary work group*, an interprofessional group that works together, but individuals work more independently than collectively. The third is an *interactive interdisciplinary team*. This final type is seen as having integrated diagnoses, team goals for patients and interdependent membership.

As noted above, these three typologies consider the level of integration of teams. Other authors, such as Jelphs and Dickinson (2008), have focused on the extent to which individuals from different disciplinary backgrounds collaborate within teams. In their work they have distinguished between *multidisciplinary*, *interdisciplinary* and *transdisciplinary* teams. They see the first type of team as one in which practitioners work in parallel, or side-by-side with each other but with little interaction; the second type of team in which practitioners work together in an interactive fashion; and the final type as one in which members work is integrated and 'transcend[s] their separate, conceptual and methodological orientations' (p. 13). The authors go on to note that this final type of team can be regarded as the highest form of teamwork.

While these typologies offer some useful ways of understanding the nature of different forms of teamwork, they also have limitations. For example, Katzenbach and Smith have compounded team performance and team type, as their descriptions of 'potential', 'real' and 'high performance' essentially describe team performance rather than different categories of teamwork. In contrast, Drinka and Clark have provided typologies which offer descriptions of different forms of disciplinarity within teams/groups. Furthermore, most typologies presented above have confused different types of 'teamwork' with different forms of interprofessional work such as collaboration and coordination. For example, Bruce's description of a nominal team arguably operates in the manner which is more like a network – a loosely connected group who interact on an episodic basis.

In general, these typologies provide a rather normative and linear understanding of teamwork – where teams may 'progress' from a state of poor functioning to a higher level of performance. In practice, interprofessional teamwork is more complex, and will vary on each of the key elements listed in Table 3.1. Indeed, there seems to be an assumption that teams operating at the 'lower ends' of these varying typologies (e.g. convenient teams, pseudo teams) need to strive to reach their upper ends to function like 'committed teams' or 'real teams'. Such an assumption overlooks the pragmatics of real world teamwork.

Contingency approach

Given the limitations of these typologies, we argue that a *contingency approach* is more useful. This approach takes into account the elements listed in Table 3.1: shared team identity, clear roles/goals, interdependence, integration, shared responsibility as well as our notion of *team tasks*. Each of these elements can be viewed as a continuum along which a particular team can be placed, for example, from having a weak team identity to having a strong, shared team identity. Teams may vary in their location along each of these dimensions independently – a team that has a strong shared team identity may, at the same time, have more loosely integrated work practices. This approach does not view teams and teamworking as moving along a linear, hierarchical spectrum from 'weak' to 'strong'. Rather, it suggests a more complex and nuanced picture of teamwork in which teams need to be matched to the purpose they are intended to serve as well as their local needs. For some purposes, greater shared responsibility among team members may be important while for other purposes it may not be so. In designing and organising teams, it may be useful to consider what configuration of each of these elements would best address or match the local goals that the team is being established to fulfil.

Given this approach, in which teams think about their purpose and also how they can respond to local needs, we argue that teamwork is only one of the forms of interprofessional work which could be considered. Other forms are collaboration, coordination and networking. Depending on local need, these forms of interprofessional work may be more effective than a teamwork approach. Figure 3.1 outlines how we have distinguished between four main types of interprofessional work.

As Figure 3.1 shows, we have located interprofessional teamwork in the centre because it can be viewed as the most 'focused' of activities with high levels of interdependence, integration and shared responsibility. The other approaches to interprofessional work – collaboration, coordination and networking – are

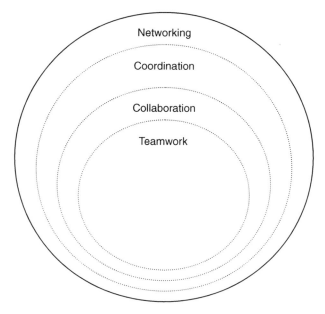

Figure 3.1 Differing forms of interprofessional work.

increasingly broader activities with reduced levels of interdependence, integration and so on.

While this typology is tentative in nature, and needs empirical testing before we can be confident of its applicability to real life, it begins to indicate how different types of interprofessional work can be considered contingent on the nature of responding to local need. Below we provide further details of these different forms of interprofessional work.

Teamwork

As noted above, teamwork encompasses a number of core elements including, but not restricted to, shared team identity, clarity, interdependence, integration, shared responsibility and team tasks which are generally unpredictable, urgent and complex. Examples of this type of interprofessional work include intensive care teams and emergency department/room teams (e.g. Piquette *et al.*, 2009a, 2009b). Box 3.2 provides an illustration of this type of interprofessional work.

Box 3.2   An example of interprofessional teamwork.

Based in an emergency department, a small team of nurses, physicians, pharmacists and respiratory therapists work together to meet the needs of patients, who arrive unpredictably with a range of acute conditions which need immediate attention. The team functions in an integrative fashion, with each member interacting and communicating to perform their profession-specific tasks in a clear and timely manner. Team members often come together to debrief and reflect when they encounter a complex clinical episode. Over their time together, trust and mutual support has grown between members, who often socialise with one another in the evenings. Consequently, the members feel a strong sense of membership with their team.

Collaboration

Collaboration is a 'looser' form of interprofessional work. It differs from teamwork in that shared identity and integration of individuals are less important. However, it is similar to teamwork in requiring shared accountability between individuals, some interdependence between individuals, clarity of roles/goals and team tasks which are generally a little more unpredictable, less urgent and complex. Examples of this type of interprofessional work can be found in primary care and general medical settings (e.g. Delva *et al.*, 2008) (also see Box 3.3).

Coordination

Coordination as a form of interprofessional work is similar to collaboration in terms of shared identity. However, integration and interdependence is less

---

Box 3.3   An example of interprofessional collaboration.

Within a large general medical ward groups of physicians, nurses, occupational therapists, physiotherapists, pharmacists and social workers practice together to provide care to an increasingly ageing local population with a range
of acute and social conditions. In general, ward members work well together,
they communicate, albeit briefly, when they need to, over patient care issues.
Nevertheless, apart from undertaking this form of ward-based interaction and
a weekly interprofessional meeting, the professionals who work in this setting
do not feel they have a shared team identity. Many mention that apart from
periodic interprofessional interaction to meet patients' needs, there is little further communication. On occasions though, the group shares a joke or a box of
chocolates given by a patient about to be discharged.

---

crucial. Team tasks are more predictable and less urgent than collaboration. Coordination is similar to collaboration in that it does require some shared accountability between individuals and clarity of roles/tasks/goals. This type of interprofessional work has been outlined by Gittell *et al.* (2000) who used the notion of
'relational coordination', which requires frequent, timely and accurate communication among providers to coordinate care. Examples of this type of interprofessional work can be found in the case management literature which describes how
individuals, usually called case managers, coordinate the work of the other team
members (see Box 3.4).

Box 3.4   An example of interprofessional coordination.

Based in a community mental health organisation groups of psychiatrists,
psychiatric nurses, social workers and occupational therapists work together
to provide care to individuals with moderate mental health conditions. These
professionals meet once a week to briefly review and discuss their shared
work. Other than this meeting, these individuals work in parallel with one
another.

Networking

A networking relationship is one in which shared team identity, clarity of
roles/goals, interdependence, integration and shared responsibility are less essential. Tasks are also more predictable and non-urgent. Networks can be virtual, in
the sense that none of the members meet face-to-face, but communicate by use of
the internet (e.g. email or computer conferencing). Øvretveit (1997, p. 271) notes
that 'networks are informal arrangements with a changing membership', highlighting that individuals may move through these networks as the need arises

for specific skills or expertise. Examples of this type of interprofessional work include networks of clinicians who share information on adverse reactions to drugs, or groups of clinicians who meet to discuss the application of clinical guidelines across a number of institutions (see Box 3.5).

Box 3.5   An example of an interprofessional network.

Based in a public health department, a group of nurses, nutritionists and physicians who have developed a mutual interest in food safety and food-borne illness have begun to meet once a month to discuss and debate this subject. They often email one another in-between meetings to keep each other updated on any new developments in this field.

An adaptive interprofessional team

In Box 3.6 we have considered how a team might function if it could employ each of these differing types of interprofessional work, as outlined in Boxes 3.2–3.5. In doing so, the team would essentially function in an *adaptive* manner – changing to the different needs of the patient.

Box 3.6   An adaptive interprofessional team.

Based within an acute care setting, the geriatric falls team consists of a range of professions including dietetics, medicine, nursing, occupational therapy, physiotherapy, speech and language therapy, and social work. They work together to provide care to older adults who suffer injury due to a fall. This includes medical care, rehabilitation and community liaison. The team's approach to care is one in which they regularly communicate in order to adapt to the needs of their patients and their families. They therefore shift seamlessly from providing medical care (involving physicians and nurses), to rehabilitation care (involving dietetics, physiotherapy and speech and language therapy) to resettlement care (involving occupational therapy and social workers). As a result of frequent team discussion and negotiation, the team work together in a manner where they shift between different kinds of interprofessional work depending on the patient need. They switch from teamwork in the initial admission when patients can need intensive input from the team to collaboration and coordination in the latter stages of their care where patient needs are focused upon rehabilitation and returning home.

As indicated in Box 3.6, an adaptive team depends on a contingency approach in which they adapt the nature of their work – from teamwork to collaboration to networking back to teamwork – depending upon changes in local needs.

Comparing typologies of teamworking

We now consider how our typology of interprofessional work (Figure 3.1) relates to the team typologies described by Bruce (1980), Katzenbach and Smith (1993), Drinka and Clark (2000) and Jelphs and Dickinson (2008). Table 3.2 outlines how these authors' descriptions of varying types of team fit into the categories of teamwork, collaboration, coordination and networking.

Table 3.2   Making sense of different teamwork typologies.

| | Author/typology | | | |
Our typology	Bruce	Katzenbach and Smith	Drinka and Clark	Jelphs and Dickenson
Teamwork	Committed teams	High performance, real, potential teams	Interactive interdisciplinary teams	Transdisciplinary teams
Collaboration	Convenient teams	Pseudo teams	Multidisciplinary work groups	Interdisciplinary teams
Coordination				Multidisciplinary teams
Networking	Nominal teams	Working groups	Ad hoc task groups	

As Table 3.2 indicates, these team typologies do fit reasonably well into our different categories of interprofessional work. Table 3.2 also helps to illustrate a possible misuse of the term 'team' in the literature. As we have discussed above, for us, teamwork is one specific form of interprofessional work that involves a certain set of characteristics, in contrast with other forms. In order to avoid confusion, we recommend that the term 'teamwork' should not be employed as a generic, all encompassing term.

Factors which affect team performance

As well as describing the various characteristics of teamwork, the literature also outlines the key elements that contribute to team performance (i.e. how well a team functions). Hackman (1983), for instance, writing from an organisational perspective, offers a model in which he describes five conditions that influence team performance:

- Collectively, the team has a compelling direction for its work
- The team's structure facilitates collaborative work. For example, there is open communication between members of the team
- The organisational context within which the team works is supportive
- The team has access to hands-on coaching to help members maximise their performance within the work circumstances
- Members collectively responsible for the teamwork.

As can be seen, these conditions relate closely to the key elements of teamworking described above.

Writing some years later, Hackman (1990) stated that team performance also requires continuity of team membership, collective contribution to members' well-being and professional growth and appropriate team composition (i.e. team size). In this model, team norms (e.g. the shared ideas and practices employed by the team) are also important elements of an effective (or high performing) team.

For West (1994), team performance is linked to three key factors. The first is 'task effectiveness' and is focused on the extent to which the team is successful in achieving its task-related objectives. The second is 'mental health' and encompasses notions of well-being, growth and development of team members. The final factor is 'team viability' which focuses on the notion of how probable it is that the team will continue to work together and function effectively. Unlike the approach proposed by Hackman, this framework does not explicitly consider contextual factors, such as organisational support, or the extent to which the team has a shared objective. However, these factors are to some extent implicit within the elements of task effectiveness, mental health and team viability.

Borrill et al. (2001) regard team performance as linked to the Donabedian (1966) approach of input–process–output. They state that team inputs are composed of elements such as environment, organisational context and team composition. Team process is seen as consisting of leadership, clarity of objectives, participation, task orientation, support for innovation, decision-making and communication/integration. Team outputs are centred around clinical outcomes/quality of care, innovation, cost-effectiveness, team member mental health and team member turnover.

According to Heinemann and Zeiss (2002), team performance comprises four elements. The first, context, includes the relationship that the team shares with its host institution, as influenced by environment, organisational structures and finances. The second, domain and structure, focuses on the membership, composition and organisation of the team. Third, process, is concerned with how the team is shaped by communication patterns, how power and influence affects the team, and the evolving team relations. The final element, productivity, considers the impact of the team in terms of what they are able to achieve.

Lemieux-Charles and McGuire (2006) have, more recently, offered an integrated team performance model designed to help understand factors that influence team function and the ability of teams to perform effectively. In this approach, effectiveness is achieved by obtaining clearly defined measures which are identified by considering responses to the following questions:

- At the practice level – what is the task of the team? What are the specific features that distinguish the task carried out by the team? What is the composition of the team (i.e. size, age, gender)? What processes exist to enhance teamwork? What are the psychosocial traits of the team (i.e. team norms, team cohesion)?

- At the organisational level – what is the organisational context in which the team exists (i.e. resources available, organisational support)?
- At the systems level – what is the social and political context related to teams (i.e. systemic factors)?

Table 3.3 provides a summary and synthesis of these authors' work, highlighting key overarching factors that may influence team performance.

Table 3.3 Summary of factors influencing team performance.

Author	Factor	Key factors
Hackman	Team process (e.g. team membership) Organisational context (e.g. support for team) Team structure (size of team) Team outputs (e.g. quality 'products')	
West	Team effectiveness Mental health of the team Team viability	
Heinemann and Ziess	Team structure (composition of team) Organisational context Team process (e.g. communication) Team productivity (e.g. impact)	Organisational context Team processes Team structure Team outputs
Borrill and colleagues	Team inputs (e.g. environment, size) Team processes (e.g. decision making) Team outputs (e.g. cost-effectiveness, member mental health)	
Lemieux-Charles and McGuire	Practice factors (e.g. team tasks) Organisational context Systems factors (e.g. politics)	

As Table 3.3 indicates, the descriptions of team performance proposed in this work share a number of common elements that can be grouped together in the following areas: organisational context, team processes, team structure and team outputs. Although these models have usefully captured key team and organisational factors, only Lemieux-Charles and McGuire has acknowledged the influence of wider systems factors on teamwork. This neglect of context level factors is problematic. While the explanation may lie in the largely social-psychological background of the majority of teamwork authors, the result is that a number of these models overlook the impact on team performance of factors such as members' gender, ethnicity and socio-economic status.

Table 3.3 also raises a question about the notion of team performance. For example, should one measure team performance on the basis of whether the goals or outputs of the team are achieved or whether the team, in itself, works well together? Should more weight be given to one of these factors over the other? Despite the obvious importance of all, the teamwork literature has traditionally focused more on reporting outputs and productivity, less on team processes.

Another concern about these descriptions is that the factors that influence a team's performance will depend upon a range of other issues such as clinical setting, nature of the clinical work and the type of patient care delivered.

Teamwork in non-health care settings

Having explored how interprofessional teamwork has been conceptualised, we now examine how teamwork approaches developed in non-care settings resonate (or not) with those in health and social care. In doing so, we question the assumption which underpins the work of a number of authors writing about health and social care teamwork who often draw strong parallels between these settings. Through discussion of the nature of teamwork undertaken in three non-care settings – the air-travel industry, industrial quality improvement and team sports – we attempt to establish the extent they 'fit' within an interprofessional health and social care context.

While concepts and metaphors from teamwork studies in industry and sports settings are often cited in the health and social care literature (see below), published empirical work on teams does not generally cross disciplinary boundaries. Box 3.7 details a rare study in which Larson and LaFasto interviewed individuals from a range of teams based in private and public settings to help establish some cross-cutting teamwork issues.

Box 3.7 A comparison of teamwork based in private and public funded settings.

Larson and LaFasto (1989) interviewed 31 individuals working in a variety of teams drawn from a range of contexts including industry, sports and the armed forces to explore team members' perceptions about the elements contributing to effective team performance. Their analysis indicated eight core characteristics: a clear, elevating goal; a focus on outcomes; competent members; unified commitment; a collaborative climate; standards of excellence; external support and recognition; and clear leadership. The authors go on to report that a key element of team performance is a collaborative climate, which consisted of honesty, openness, consistency and respect. Larson and LaFasto also found a number of problems which could impede the development of a collaborative climate and team performance. They pointed out that there was a need to balance the autonomy of team members with approaches to ensuring their involvement in the team. Other team-based problems included the need to ensure support and recognition for team efforts; difficulties in maintaining shared trust; as well as the need to restrict the development of cliques or subgroups.

While the study in Box 3.7 provides a helpful insight into a range of possible factors that may affect teamwork and team performance across a variety of settings, the reliance on interview data alone means that the findings generated from this work are based on individuals' impressions and perceptions of teamwork and not on field observations of teamwork in action. As a result, it is difficult to assess the extent to which such descriptions reflect the reality of teamwork in practice, as individuals' recollections of the factors affecting team performance may be influenced by both social desirability and recall biases. Nonetheless, it is notable that the factors identified in this study mirror many of those included in the models presented above (see Table 3.3).

Aircraft crews

One of the foremost efforts by the aviation community to develop safe teams is the training programme known as Crew (or Cockpit) Resource Management (CRM) (Helmreich *et al.*, 1999). CRM originated in 1979 from work undertaken by the National Aeronautics and Space Administration (NASA) on improving aircraft safety. NASA identified that the primary cause of the majority of aviation accidents was human error, and that the main problems were failures of communication, leadership and decision-making in the cockpit. CRM training was subsequently adopted by the aviation industry. It is now a mandated requirement for commercial aircrews working under most regulatory bodies worldwide.

The CRM approach relies upon integrated training in communication, disclosure and teamwork behaviours that facilitate the balanced management of all resources required for safe flight. In initiating this new approach, airlines have moved away from training the individual pilot to training the entire crew. This is based on the recognition that safety and good performance are not just the focus of the captain, but the entire crew. Central to this approach to safety improvement has been attention in establishing a shared understanding of how all members of the crew perceive a situation, their role in it and their interactions with other crew members.

This approach appears to have been successful in helping to reduce accidents on large aircraft (Salas *et al.*, 2008). Flights are now governed by explicit, detailed written procedures which cover almost all situations and problems. Tasks and their allocation to different members of the crew are clear. Small flight crews are trained to ensure that each member's work is carried out in a highly collaborative fashion. Processes are monitored to detect errors and neither fear of blame nor the professional hierarchy of the cockpit are allowed to interrupt information flow or problem-solving. Smooth operation of these systems is eased by the following factors:

- Defined boundaries to the task (preparation, takeoff, flight, landing)
- A fixed crew for the duration of each flight
- Simple shared goals to which the crew is committed

- Close proximity of crew members
- Guaranteed communication links via earphones and microphones
- Regular re-training by use of high fidelity simulation learning methods.

While a CRM approach has yielded some useful gains within the aviation industry, its impact on other domains has yet to be established. Recently, Salas *et al.* (2006) undertook a review of published accounts of CRM training to determine its effectiveness within a number of fields such as the maritime industry. While they found that the training generally produced positive reactions from trainees, its impact on knowledge acquisition and behaviour was mixed. The authors conclude that at present it is not possible to ascertain whether CRM can improve an organisation's safety, outside of aircraft crews.

Application to health and social care

Despite a paucity of evidence, CRM has been widely adopted by many health care organisations (e.g. Risser *et al.*, 1999; Sexton *et al.*, 2000; Pizzi *et al.*, 2001). In many respects, this approach has a good fit with a number of care settings such as emergency rooms, intensive care units and operating rooms/theatres. In these locations, the team takes responsibility for the patient's defined problems and deals with them in priority order, under the leadership of a physician or surgeon. There are (usually) standardised procedures, protocols and algorithms that can be followed. However, with more than 90% of health and social care provided in less structured, low intensity settings like clinicians' offices, patients' homes, hospital outpatient departments or inpatient wards (Green *et al.*, 2001), the applicability of CRM may be more limited.

The differences between health and social care and the airline industry also extend to the nature of tasks. While most patients have common diagnoses, every case is rendered unique by the interaction of multiple problems and with personal and social situations. As a result, a standardised CRM approach to delivering care in these situations is inappropriate. Indeed, the central challenge for clinicians is that patient care tasks can be complex, evolving and difficult to specify. Moreover, with severely ill patients, there is variability in the kind of teamwork they need, as we previously discussed in this chapter. Variability is also linked to where the patients are in their care trajectory. The complexity in a single patient hospital stay may, for example, fluctuate back and forth over time in terms of medical need in the early days to social need in the latter days and back again to medical care if an unforeseen problem occurs.

Given that evidence for the effects of CRM (outside of aviation) remains limited, any application to a health and social care setting should be undertaken with caution. Ideally, it should be preceded by a careful assessment of the relevance of the model to the 'problem' it is intended to address and implementation should be combined with careful evaluation (see Chapter 7).

Quality improvement teams

The focus on industrial quality improvement (QI) and teamwork emerged in the 1940s in response to the need for high-quality, low-cost materials for World War II. The QI approach was subsequently popularised in the Japanese automobile manufacturing industry in the 1960s and 1970s. The QI movement rests upon three core principles:

- Continuous efforts to achieve stable and predictable results (i.e. reduce process variation) are key to success and productivity
- Manufacturing and business processes have characteristics that can be measured, analysed, improved and controlled
- Achieving sustained QI requires commitment and collaboration across the organisation from management to front-line workers.

On the basis of these principles, which were subsequently informed theoretically by the work of Argyris and Schön (1978), a number of broadly similar QI approaches emerged, starting with continuous quality improvement (CQI) and total quality management (TQM).

Other quality approaches to gain popularity include Quality Circles, Kaizen, Lean Methods and Six Sigma (e.g. Blumenthal and Kilo, 1998; Barry et al., 2002; Radnor et al., 2006; Sherman, 2006). Quality Circles were, for example, initially developed to help teams of workers in the automobile manufacturing industry identify and solve problems as they occurred at an individual stage in the production line. However, as most quality problems were found to span, not one, but many points in the production process, a boarder Kaizen approach was devised. Kaizen utilises multifunctional production teams to work to continuously improve quality and productivity across the entire process, rather than at an individual point.

Application to health and social care

Supported by influential organisations such as the Institute for Healthcare Improvement (IHI) and the Joint Commission for Accreditation of Healthcare Organizations (JCAHQ), QI principles have been widely employed in the US over the past decade or so among a growing variety of health and social care providers. This expansion has also been witnessed in a number of other countries' health and social care systems, including Australia, Canada and the UK, who have primarily adopted CQI and TQM approaches in their work (e.g. Gazarian et al., 2001; Treadwell et al., 2002; Wilcock et al., 2002; Yealy et al., 2004).

The use of QI approaches within health and social care context can be problematic. As QI approaches are rooted in private sector organisations whose aim it is to offer a relatively limited range of services and products, with a narrow range of variability in quality, at a competitive cost to consumers who can choose among many suppliers, they do not necessarily match the more variable processes of care delivery. This is not to say that there are no activities in health and social care which are amenable to QI processes. Laundry services, laboratory specimen processing and catering, for example, can more easily be organised in a more standardised, efficient and reliable fashion. But providing care, as we outlined in Chapters 1 and 2, involves a range of complex professional, economic and organisational factors. In addition, unlike consumers, patients are usually unique, with differing co-morbidities and social conditions, different values and personal support systems, all which challenge the ethos of QI. In addition, patients are seldom in a position to select the services they receive – they generally access services which are offered in their locale. Furthermore, when one takes a closer examination of QI initiatives employed within health and social care, they rely on the assumption that professionals can easily perform as high functioning teams, and that these teams can easily overcome simple process flaws to improve their service organisation and enhance the quality of care they deliver. Indeed, little attention is paid to attempting to improve the quality of team performance or the interprofessional team processes within most QI initiatives. Moreover, the evidence base for the use of QI initiatives within health and social care settings is very limited due to the absence of many high-quality studies, as a recent review undertaken by Vest and Gamm (2009) reported.

Sports teams

Notions of teams and teamwork in the public consciousness are often linked to sports, with these groups being seen as 'ideal' teams. Football, rugby, hockey and basketball teams all require high levels of teamwork to succeed. As well as having talent to play as an individual, it is argued that sports team members need to be effective team players, who can interact with and react to their colleagues as well as to anticipate their movements on the field of play.

Application to health and social care

While successful sports teams are commonly regarded as representing an ideal form of team, one needs to be aware of the limited nature this comparison has with interprofessional teams. For example, in sports, the ball has no agency – it is kicked or hit rather than cared for and is highly replaceable. Also, health and social care teams have no attached coaches, physiotherapists or physicians, whose primary role it is to watch the game and see who is playing well, suggest where improvements to teamwork can be made and provide care for team members' physical and psychological well-being.

The primary purpose of a sports team is simple – to score more goals, tries or points than their opponent. The purpose of health and social care teams is far more complex. Such teams need to provide high quality, error-free, individualised care to a large number of patients on a daily basis. Some of whom are severely ill, may have multiple clinical problems and may not be able to communicate in the same language, all of which makes providing care far more complicated and demanding.

To press the analogy of the sports team in health and social care slightly further, in a typical hospital, one can imagine a field with some 1000 players (professionals) and 800 balls (patients) and an infinite number of nets (treatments), or a net that is moving for each ball all the time (e.g. as treatment moves from general medicine to palliative care). Indeed, the players have to interact with other players in other fields (institutions such as primary care or specialist referral centres) as well as with a wide range of other interested parties – quality monitoring bodies, patients' families and professional associations. Such comparisons to health care are therefore highly problematic.

Conclusions and implications

While teamwork approaches from the air-travel, quality and sports industries provide some interesting ideas about how teams function, their application to health and social care is limited, as such approaches fail to pay attention to the complexities involved in working together in an interprofessional care setting.

Although the definitions, typologies and models presented above offer insights into different dimensions and functions of teams, they have their limitations. This literature mainly offers generic descriptions of teams and teamworking, which do not pay sufficient attention to the *interprofessional-ness* of teamwork. Given the role politics and economics played in the emergence of health and social care professions (see Chapters 4 and 5), interprofessional teamwork was founded upon imbalances of power and status. However, such issues remain largely untouched.

Furthermore, as the chapter indicated, many of the models of teamwork are also largely based upon the authors' personal conceptualisations – not empirical evidence. Although many of these models do have, on the surface, a degree of resonance, and review work has indicated that factors such as team context and team processes can have some affect on team performance (e.g. Stock, 2004; Jeffcott and Mackenzie, 2008), their explanatory abilities remain uncertain. Indeed, as we noted above, there is an assumption shared between typologies we presented above that teams should strive to move from 'lower end' team configurations to 'higher end' forms. As we argued, such a hierarchical notion overlooks the complexities of delivering care, which requires interprofessional teams to adopt a *contingency approach*, dependent upon particular needs, contextual influences and available resources.

4 A conceptual framework for interprofessional teamwork

Introduction

The chapter presents our conceptual framework for interprofessional teamwork as a way of navigating through the complex array of issues health and social care teams encounter in their everyday practice. We developed a framework comprising a number of factors which we have synthesised into four domains: relational, processual, organisational and contextual. These factors affect interprofessional teamwork in a number of different ways. In creating this framework we have attempted, where possible, to draw upon evidence-based sources. As we have previously noted, in the absence of evidence we have included work which we view as coherent, plausible and comprehensive. We describe and discuss each of these factors and their effect on interprofessional teamwork processes and outcomes. We also examine the interlinked nature of the factors, which for ease of presentation have been separated into four discrete main areas.

Our framework

Through a wide range of sources gathered for our work of implementing and evaluating interprofessional education and practice, we identified a number of salient teamwork factors which we synthesised into the following four domains:

- Relational – factors which directly affect the relationships shared by professionals such as professional power and socialisation
- Processual – factors such as space and time which affect how the work of the team is carried out across different workplace situations
- Organisational – factors that affect the local organisational environment in which the interprofessional team operates
- Contextual – factors related to the broader social, political and economic landscape in which the team is located.

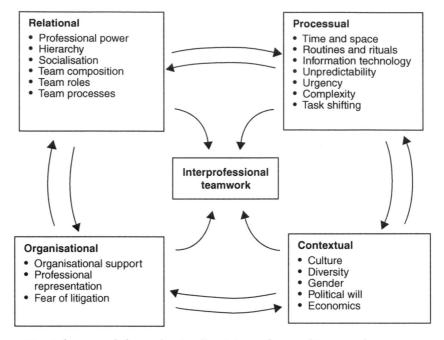

Figure 4.1   A framework for understanding interprofessional teamwork.

Figure 4.1 provides a diagrammatic representation of our framework. It outlines a number of separate factors in bullet form. As the arrows in Figure 4.1 suggest, each of these factors is linked with one domain, but has the ability to affect interprofessional teamwork in different ways. In the remainder of the chapter we discuss *how* these factors can affect (facilitate or inhibit) teamwork.

While, for simplicity, we have arranged these factors under four domains, there is some overlap between them, which we discuss later in the chapter. We should also note that although we have attempted to offer a framework which provides a comprehensive insight into a wide range of issues related to teamwork, this is not (nor could it be) an exhaustive set of factors. It is rooted within our shared interests on teamworking and so reflects our mutual interests. Therefore, in many ways this framework offers a *sociologically* informed view of interprofessional teamwork – a perspective which has been largely absent from the teamwork literature.

Relational factors

As indicated in Figure 4.1, we identified the following six relational factors: professional power, hierarchy, socialisation, team composition, team roles and team processes. Before we describe each, Box 4.1 provides an example of how a relational factor, in this case hierarchy, can affect interprofessional teamwork in a rehabilitation setting.

> **Box 4.1** Interprofessional teamwork and hierarchy.
>
> Cott (1998) examined the meanings of 'teamwork' employed by an interprofessional team who worked in a hospital-based long-term older adult care unit. Drawing upon Strauss' negotiated order perspective (see Chapter 5), she gathered interview data with team members. These data indicated the existence of two subgroups within the interprofessional team. One of the subgroups consisted of physicians, therapists and social workers who occupied a high position in the team hierarchy as they could take decisions on aspects of patient care. The other consisted of junior qualified and unqualified nursing staff who occupied lower positions in the hierarchy as they could not take such decisions. Cott also found that views of teamwork were largely dependent upon the type of work that was undertaken, as well as the position in the team hierarchy. It was reported that the subgroup of physicians, therapists and social workers collaborated in an equal fashion, discussing and agreeing on aspects of patient care. For this subgroup, teamwork was essentially viewed as vital for improving quality of care they delivered. By contrast, in the subgroup which consisted of junior qualified and unqualified staff, collaborative work was directed by a senior nurse. As a result, this subgroup did not decide how they worked together, nor did they have much direct contact with the physicians, therapists or social workers, who usually communicated with the senior nurse. In addition, this subgroup's view of teamwork rested on the notion that it simply made their job easier to undertake.

Professional power

Power is a complex phenomenon. A number of sociological perspectives have described and analysed its multiple (positive and negative) dimensions (e.g. Clegg, 1989). In relation to power among the health and social care professions, as medicine was the first health care occupation to professionalise, it secured areas of high status knowledge and expertise and so attained high levels of social status and economic reward (Freidson, 1970). Over the years medicine has successfully protected these gains to achieve the dominant position of power in relation to the other health and social care professions. When one considers the nature of medicine's power, it has the ability to influence the policymaking agenda, as well as (largely) control collaboration and care delivery processes (e.g. Fiorelli, 1988; Hugman, 1991; Gardezi et al., 2009). As a result of this dominance, it has been argued that medicine's position is *hegemonic* in nature (Gramsci, 1988). But recent developments such as the rise of consumer movements and the increasing involvement of government in care (e.g. Ferlie et al., 1996) have weakened medicine's traditional power base to some extent.

Mackay et al. (1995) have argued that engagement in interprofessional activities such as teamwork rests upon the readiness to share power. They go on to suggest that professions such as nursing and physiotherapy have a direct interest in collaborating with medicine, as it can help enhance their own influence over the care delivery process. Exploring this issue of equality within interprofessional teams, Gibbon (1999) points out that notions of power sharing between professions may *mask* the underlying power differentials:

> In reality team members do not share equality [. . .] this is part of the rhetoric of teamwork and is misleading at best, and patronising at worse. (p. 248)

When one considers the effects of power and the ability to influence decisions, behaviours and actions, according to Foucault (1978) one needs also to be aware of resistance to power. Resistance in interprofessional teams can come in different forms – passive (apathy towards other team members and collective work) and active, such as committing errors or the spoilage of shared projects (Gelmon *et al.*, 2000; Delva *et al.*, 2008). In our work we found resistance was usually played out in passive forms, such as non-attendance at team meetings (Reeves and Lewin, 2004).

Despite the inequalities of power which exist, and the friction that can be caused by such imbalances, interprofessional relationships need to be *managed* on a daily basis between practitioners in order to deliver patient care in a collaborative fashion. Chapter 6 outlines a number of interventions which may help engage team members in a range of activities designed to develop shared agreement around their daily collaborative work.

Hierarchy

Division of labour within many private and public sector organisations is hierarchical – a vertical arrangement whereby individuals with seniority have the authority to supervise the work of their juniors. The development and maintenance of hierarchies often rests upon social, economic and political inequalities. When one considers the nature of hierarchy between the health and social care professions, there are two main dimensions. First, as noted above, the professionalisation processes which occurred between the professions resulted in an emergence of an interprofessional hierarchy in which medicine occupies the dominant position. Second, each of the professions is internally organised along hierarchies based on experience and seniority – the more of each an individual has, the higher the position in the professional hierarchy they are usually located.

Hierarchical structures can have an inhibiting effect on interprofessional teamwork (e.g. Sexton *et al.*, 2000; Di Palma, 2004). For example, they can disempower students and junior staff from making potentially valuable suggestions to their senior colleagues, as well as adversely affect engagement in interprofessional teamwork (see Box 4.1).

Relations between different interprofessional teams can also be impeded by hierarchy. Higher status teams, for example those in which members publish research, can achieve a high profile. As a result, their members are more likely to secure better access to organisational resources than colleagues who work in lower profile, lower status teams.

Hierarchies can be helpful. Such arrangements can ensure that more experienced staff are able to provide support to junior staff in their clinical practice. Nevertheless, attention is needed to ensure that hierarchical arrangements do not reinforce traditional notions of dominance or inhibit the free flow of communication between team members, as a recent study by Mahmood-Yousuf *et al.* (2008) on teamwork within a palliative care setting indicated.

Socialisation

Professional socialisation is a process in which individuals acquire the norms, values and attitudes associated with a particular professional group. As a result, certain patterns of language, dress, demeanour and behaviours are assumed and emphasised through ongoing interactions with peers and more senior members of the profession (Clark, 1997).

Sociological studies by authors such as Becker *et al.* (1961), and more recently Sinclair (1997), have indicated that professional socialisation usually results in individuals strongly associating and identifying with their professional group. Often, the socialisation leads to the adoption of a 'closed' professional identity with its own behaviours, language, values and attitudes, which can mean that engagement in interprofessional collaboration is regarded as a low priority. Indeed, Blane (1991) argued that socialisation results in individuals whose 'primary loyalty is to their own profession' (p. 231) and an *inward looking* stance which can impede efforts to engage in interprofessional teamwork.

Processes of professional socialisation often occur before an individual has entered their selected profession, often through the media. As Reeves and Pryce (1998) reported in their study of first year medical, nursing and dental students, many entered their respective professional course with pre-existing notions of traditional professional stereotypes and hierarchies. The effects of professional socialisation can therefore be profound. Indeed, as indicated above, they can lead to the development of values and attitudes which may profoundly undermine teamwork.

Team composition

Composition, in terms of size and membership, is a key element in how a team functions. There is some evidence which indicates that teams who have over ten members encounter more difficulties working together than smaller teams (e.g. Williams and Laungani, 1999). West (1994) has argued that a team which has over 25 members can be regarded as a small organisation, given the width of individuals' needs, demands and interests. Naturally, the larger the team, the more difficult it will be to schedule meetings, coordinate members' tasks and agree upon a joint approach. It has also been noted that within large teams, subgroups can emerge (Douglas, 2000). This can occur when a small number of members who hold ideas that diverge from the majority work together in an exclusionary fashion.

Handy (1999, p. 155) argues that large teams may have some advantages in terms of a greater amount of 'talent, skills and knowledge'. He goes on to note, however, that there is usually more absenteeism and lower morale in larger teams; as members generally meet less and have limited opportunity for developing a team rapport.

The nature of team membership, in particular representation of different professional groups, can also affect function. For example, a community mental health team populated by many nurses and social workers can be overwhelming for the occupational therapist and psychologist who tend to operate as the only representative of their profession (Reeves *et al.*, 2006).

Team roles

The formation and preservation of clear professional roles is seen as an essential element for effective interprofessional team relations and team performance (e.g. West and Markiowicz, 2004). Clear roles help define the nature of each team members' tasks, responsibilities and scope of practice. Given the bounded nature of each profession's scope of practice, there is a need to monitor and protect their areas of expertise. Clear roles within a team help ensure that problems around professional boundary infringement are avoided. Nevertheless, on occasions teams work in a *generic* manner where different team members share roles. For example, in remote rural areas, limited numbers of practitioners means that there is a need to regularly work across traditional professional boundaries. However, generic working can generate friction between team members as they are unclear about their respective professional roles (e.g. Booth and Hewison, 2002; Stark *et al.*, 2002).

A key team role is that of the team leader (Martin and Rogers, 2004). A useful definition of an interprofessional team leader has been offered by Cook (2003), who regards them as individuals who influence others through their ability to motivate, take decisions and encourage innovation. A range of different leadership models can be found in the teamwork literature. In essence, they employ a continuum in which leaders can be placed somewhere between the extremes of autocratic or democratic approaches. Bass (1997), for example, argues there are two essential types of leaders, 'transactional' and 'transformational'. The former adopt an authoritative approach, tend to work in isolation from the team and make decisions without including team members. By contrast, the latter adopts a democratic approach, works flexibly with members and promotes creative problem-solving within the team.

Leadership within interprofessional teams can be problematic. Separate professional responsibilities and different lines of management of members mean that identifying a single leader can be difficult (Øvretveit, 1993; Norman and Peck, 1999). Also, leadership is complicated as the team may need to change leaders when the care needs of their patients change. For example, in general medicine, a patient's medical needs may be straightforward and met quickly, but their need for social care may become very complex. Team leadership, therefore, needs to shift from medicine to social work, as this change in patient care occurs. Although as we discussed above, medical dominance of the care process may mean this does not routinely happen.

Team processes

Team processes are multidimensional. We see them as including the following elements: communication, team stability, team emotions, trust and respect, team-building activities, conflict and humour.

Communication

Communication within interprofessional teams occurs in a variety of verbal and non-verbal forms. It can take place synchronously or asynchronously via the use of information technology (IT). Open and free-flowing communication between team members is important to their ability to deliver care in an effective fashion. Indeed, as we previously noted, miscommunication among professions has been the single most frequent cause of adverse clinical events. This can result in problems ranging from delays in treatment to medication errors to wrong site surgery. Effective communication can be difficult to achieve as these processes can be impeded by interprofessional tensions caused by hierarchy, socialisation and power differences. Communication can also be impeded when team members work in different locations at different times of the day or at night.

Team emotions

The emotional attachments individuals have with their teams can be influential. Writing from a psychodynamic perspective, Zagier Roberts (1994) argues that the membership of a team normally carries a distinct set of emotions. Often individuals can become very attached to the team they work within. Normally, this occurs because they have developed a deep commitment to their team as they find membership to be an emotionally rewarding experience.

Van Maanen and Kunda (1989) note that given the ebbs and flows of an individual's emotions within a team, the notion of 'emotional labour' is useful to consider. Miller *et al.* (2008) explored how emotional labour affected interprofessional relations within an acute care setting. They found that nurses were strongly influenced by emotion in their interprofessional work. The establishment and maintenance of a nursing *esprit de corps*, friction with physicians and the failure of other team members to acknowledge their nursing work were all elements that affected their emotions and their readiness to engage in interprofessional work.

Trust and respect

The development of trust and respect within an interprofessional team is another important relational element. In many ways, trust and respect are built through shared experience, particularly during instances in which team members can demonstrate their technical skill and professional competence. Often a new member is not trusted until their abilities are proven (e.g. Rice Simpson *et al.*, 2006; McCallin and Bamford, 2007). High levels of trust and respect, usually based on stable team membership (see below), can allow team members to work together in a close, integrated fashion (Ohlinger *et al.*, 2003; Institute of Medicine, 2004b). An absence of these qualities can, however, be problematic. As Walby *et al.* (1994) found in their interviews with 127 doctors and 135 nurses, a lack of respect was reported as a key source of interprofessional conflict between these two professions across a range of clinical settings. In addition, poor levels of trust and respect contributed to poor knowledge of one another, limited commitment to shared team goals and fragmented interprofessional communication.

Humour

The use of humour in teams can play a number of important functions. It can be employed to emphasise existing rules and boundaries, reinforce power imbalances or ease interprofessional tension. Griffiths (1998) explored the role and influence of humour within two community mental health teams. Both consisted of physicians, nurses, social workers and occupational therapists. Audio recordings of team meetings revealed that humour was used as a way of 'letting off steam' (p. 892) in relation to the general stresses and strains of working together. It was also a mechanism that helped team members support one another in their work with patients who had serious mental health problems. In addition, the study revealed that team members used humorous comments to 'signal their unease about certain referrals' (p. 884) to the team leader or to question a course of action with a patient. Often this resulted in a change to planned action by the team leader.

Conflict

As we discussed above, conflict between team members can arise due to a number of relational factors. While interprofessional conflict can be problematic to team relations and team performance, it can also have positive effects. West (1994), for example, states that conflict between members can be a source of innovation and 'a source of excellence, quality and creativity' (p. 71). Nevertheless, any conflict needs to be well handled within a team. If not, it can become damaging to interprofessional interactions and general team function.

It has also been found that an absence of conflict or friction within a team can develop a phenomenon termed 'groupthink' – where there is a lack of disagreement and debate between team or group members (Janis, 1982). In such teams, rather than seek opposing views and opinions, members prefer to focus upon reaching agreement and consensus. This can mean that teams fail to consider the range of possibilities around how they solve a particular problem. Recent work which explored the nature of decision-making in an interprofessional planning group indicated that a lack of critical analysis due to a shared need for consensus and agreement, contributed to the development of groupthink (Reeves, 2008).

Team stability

The stability of team membership can have an effect on interprofessional relations. The literature has suggested that a health care team with stable membership, is likely to perform in an effective manner as, over time, members will have been able to develop mutual understanding and trust with one another (e.g. West and Slater, 1996; Gair and Hartery, 2001). Nevertheless, as Vanclay (1996) noted in health and social care, achieving stability can be difficult. There may be a regular turnover of staff which can mean that there is rarely sufficient time for team members to 'know each other well [and] foster a teamwork ethos' (p. 1).

Individual willingness

Willingness to work in a collaborative manner cannot simply be assumed. An individual needs to be willing to engage in teamwork. As Henneman *et al.* (1995, p. 106) point out, 'only the person involved ultimately determines whether or not collaboration occurs'. As we noted above, individuals can and do employ a range of subtle strategies to resist the influence of others to participate in activities they do not wish to undertake. Willingness to engage (or not) in teamwork can involve a number of factors. As Skjørshammer (2001) found, engagement in collaboration depended on a number of elements including the nature of the care task, its perceived urgency and need for interdependence between professions. Therefore, if an individual clinician felt that a care task had both low urgency and low interdependence, they may avoid engaging in interprofessional work.

Team-building

Regular team-building activities aimed at enhancing collaborative processes can help teams improve their performance. Typically, such activities include a range of interactive learning opportunities (e.g. workshops, retreats and, more recently, online sessions) which aim to develop and enhance teamwork attitudes, knowledge, skills and behaviours (also see Chapter 6). The use of team reflection activities can, for instance, be helpful for team function. West (1996) argues that teams who can spend time together reflecting upon their collaborative work can develop into a 'reflexive' team. The development of a reflexive team can help ensure that members are able to adapt and respond collectively to changes they encounter. While opportunities for team-building activities are regarded as important in improving shared performance, many teams can find it difficult to undertake these types of activities. Heavy workloads and limited resources mean that they often do not have the time or funding to undertake any team-building activities.

Processual factors

As indicated in Figure 4.1, we identified the following seven processual factors: time and space, routines and rituals, IT, unpredictability, urgency, complexity and task shifting. Before we describe each, Box 4.2 provides an example of how professions' routines, as well as the spatial layout of a team's base, can affect their ability to communicate and collaborate.

Box 4.2   How routines and spatial issues affect teamwork.

Drawing upon focus group data from six primary care teams, Delva *et al.* (2008) explored members' views regarding what elements constituted a 'team' and what factors affected team effectiveness. A number of themes emerged relating to the roles and relationships of different members. Importantly, the study indicated that interprofessional communication was often impeded by two main factors. First, physician-based communication was problematic as their attendance at team meetings was poor because these meetings often conflicted with their profession-specific schedules. Second, nursing participants noted that the spatial layout of their clinic contributed to a lack of interaction between different members. As a result of these two factors, it was reported that information between team members was inconsistently shared and often incomplete in nature.

Time and space

Time and space are entwined concepts which affect interprofessional teamwork in differing ways. Both, as Durkheim (1976) observed, are social in origin, suggesting that the temporal and spatial aspects of clinical work are linked strongly to the social organisation of that work. Armstrong (1985) suggested the spatial boundaries that traditionally separate health and social care professions also serve to fragment the patient and their illness. Such fragmentation may promote profession-specific tasks and so inhibit interprofessional teamwork (e.g. Pryor, 2008). Given these challenges, attention has recently been focused on how health and social care professions can work together in more shared team spaces to help support regular interaction and communication (e.g. Grinspun, 2007).

In terms of temporal elements, despite having little idea about the 'optimum' time teams need to share in order perform in an effective manner, it is generally agreed that *more* shared time, rather than less, is needed to evolve and develop mutual understanding, trust and respect (e.g. Jaques, 1998). Of course, simply spending time together will not necessarily result in an improvement in relationships or performance. Time, therefore, needs to be considered in relation to the engagement of shared team-building activities. In addition, the use of 'informal time' (e.g. social events) can provide additional opportunities for social interaction which allow members to develop a better understanding of one another outside their formal roles.

However, increasing heavy demands on professionals' time often means they have little opportunity to focus on improving the quality of their team relations. For example, in her ethnographic study of interprofessional relationships within acute care, Allen (2002) reported that physicians and nurses often experience difficulties communicating with one another as their clinical work resulted in them being located in different parts of a hospital at different times of the day. Opportunities for face-to-face discussions with one another, and other team members were therefore limited. Such time pressures has led Engeström *et al.* (1999) to question whether the traditional ideas of 'teamwork' fit the realities of working in an interprofessional team. Teamworking could be seen more as a process of 'knotworking' in which individuals tie, untie and re-tie separate threads of activity during their brief interprofessional interactions (Engestrom *et al.* 1999) .

Routines and rituals

Routines can be seen as a course of standardised actions or procedures that are followed regularly across health and social care settings. Routines can be helpful as they provide a 'route map' for professions and institutions to follow when undertaking a variety of clinical tasks which are generally uncomplicated, stable and predictable in nature. However, Healey *et al.* (2006) warn against routines becoming over-automated and routinised, as once this occurs there is little thought and attention given to meeting the individual needs of patients and their families.

Over time, routines can become a *ritualised* feature of professional practice. While this term has been defined and used in multiple ways, Turner's (1969) definition is most useful. He regards rituals as 'dramas of social events which emphasise the importance of the event they symbolise or represent' (p. 59). This approach views rituals as performances that enact and institutionalise culturally constructed activities. Routines and rituals may serve multiple purposes both for individuals and teams, including psychological, social and protective functions; the identification of values and rules; and the negotiation of power (e.g. Strange, 1996; Helman, 2000).

Rituals have also been found to be commonplace across health care settings ranging from the organisation of surgery in the operating room (Katz, 1981) to ward rounds (Strange, 1996). Indeed, our own work (Lewin and Reeves, in review), which explored the nature of teamwork in an acute care setting, our data indicated the existence of ritualised teamworking practices. We found that weekly interprofessional meetings, which were designed to ostensibly facilitate and maintain collaboration, appeared to include little functional collaborative activity. Many professionals did not attend and few important decisions on patient care were taken. As a result, the meetings appeared to be ritualistic and served a range of other purposes, including constituting a *visible* demonstration of teamwork.

Information technology

As described in Chapter 2, the use of IT can assist communication between members of an interprofessional team. Synchronous communication (e.g. computer conferencing, web-based interactions) occurs simultaneously between members in different locations, whereas asynchronous communication (e.g. email) occurs between members in different places and at different times. As a result, IT can offer interprofessional teams with an additional means of supporting their work (e.g. Greenwood and Meyer, 2008). IT can also overcome traditional limitations related to the need for real-time interaction in a shared physical location.

An increasing number of authors have explored the use of IT for improving interprofessional teamwork. For example, Patel *et al.* (1999) described an initiative that employed email and electronic conferencing technology to overcome the traditional temporal–spatial problems related to teamwork in acute care context. More recently, Bali (2005) explored the use of IT to support effective knowledge management between different health care team members. Collectively this literature has helped show that IT can help support communication processes between team members. However, the use of IT presents a number of technological challenges (e.g. safe storage of sensitive information) and individual challenges (the need for ongoing training). Also, the loss of direct face-to-face interaction in favour of e-communication can, arguably, diminish the quality of these exchanges – as there is often still no substitute for real-time, face-to-face human communication.

Unpredictability

As we pointed out in Chapter 3, the unpredictability of clinical work that can occur in, for example, operating theatres, intensive care and trauma care units means that the need for interprofessional teamwork is crucial. However, in unpredictable environments, teamwork can be challenging. Emergency care is highly representative of an unpredictable setting – it is fast paced with a high turnover of, often, urgent work. Characteristics that can be valued by staff working in these settings can often be linked to the *buzz* of an arriving medical emergency. Annandale *et al.* (1999) observed interprofessional interactions in two busy emergency wards and found that as a result of the fast paced, often unpredictable flow of work, tension could regularly occur between team members.

In addition, with severely ill patients, unpredictability can also be found in the kind of interprofessional care they need. For example, a patient hospital stay may shift from needing medical, nursing and pharmacy input at initial admission to needing intensive occupational therapy, physiotherapy and social work input in the latter days of their stay. While trying to predict this complicated shift related to the care trajectory of patients and their interprofessional needs has been attempted by initiatives such as *Care Mapping* (e.g. Brooker, 2005), there are difficulties in making such predictions. Although one may know the general course of care, patient needs can often fluctuate back and forth over time, and up and down in terms of intensity. Therefore, the type of interprofessional work required needs to be adaptable between the professionals in order to schedule their own particular input in a timely manner (see Chapter 3).

Urgency

Like unpredictability, the urgency of the clinical work that occurs in settings such as intensive and trauma care clinics demands the use of an interprofessional teamwork approach. However, achieving an effective team performance in the face of clinical urgency can be challenging. Skjørshammer (2001), as noted above, found that hospital staff used different approaches to interprofessional collaboration depending upon the perceived urgency of a patient care task. When staff considered the urgency of care as high, they tended to work closely with their colleagues to deliver care in a team-based manner. By contrast, when they perceived urgency as low, staff would often avoid engaging in team-based care.

More recently, Piquette et al. (2009a) explored the perceptions of intensive care teams towards stress and interprofessional teamwork. They found that urgent acute medical crises affected team interactions in a number of ways. During such episodes of care delivery, terse forms of interaction occurred, which could result in divergent perceptions among the professionals about the nature and effects of their collaborative work.

Complexity

Due to a number of social, economic, organisational, technological and professional developments which have occurred in recent years (see Chapter 2), the delivery of care is becoming ever more complex. For example, the need for expanded knowledge and skills to provide care to patients with a range of conditions has resulted in increasing professional specialisation. Although specialisation allows for in-depth exploration of a patient's problems, it can add further pressures on teamwork and collaboration, as professionals need to alter traditional patterns of shared work to accommodate the evolving nature of providing specialised care. In addition, high levels of unpredictability and urgency of patient needs within acute care settings (see above) can mean that team members work together in high pressure environments, which also increases the complexity of functioning in an effective interprofessional manner.

Task shifting

One of the central effects of professionalisation within health and social care has been the development of distinctive areas of clinical knowledge and expertise which are protected from infringement from other groups (e.g. Freidson, 1970). However, a number of shifts (e.g. ageing populations, shortages in some professions such as medicine, changes in the number of hours professionals are allowed to work) have resulted in governments looking closely at how certain tasks traditionally undertaken by certain professions may be undertaken by others.

In response, a process of *task shifting* (sometimes called substitution or delegation) can occur, as one professional hands over tasks to another (Boyes, 1995). This notion of task shifting is also linked to the creation of new roles, such as the nurse practitioner and physician assistant roles (Hooker and McCaig, 2001). While the use of task shifting can help alleviate the heavy workloads of the more traditional professions, and can provide more flexible care in the face of rising demands placed on health and social care systems, there are a number of challenges. For example, the need to re-negotiate previously agreed professional legislation around roles and responsibilities can be complex. In addition, as Scholes and Vaughan (2002) found in their study on the effects of task shifting between nursing and medicine in interprofessional teams in the UK, careful negotiation was required between individuals when attempting to expand the nursing role into the area of medicine, as sensitivities related to professional boundary protectionism arose. Furthermore, task shifting in the form of delegation can reinforce the hierarchical position of professions, as there is a handover of what can be perceived as 'low status' tasks. This can also threaten the professional status of one profession in relation to another.

Organisational factors

Figure 4.1 outlined three key organisational factors: organisational support, professional representation and fear of litigation. Box 4.3 provides an insight into why organisational support is a central factor to the performance of interprofessional teams.

Box 4.3   The role of organisational support in teamwork.

Xyrichis and Lowton (2008) reviewed the interprofessional teamwork literature in primary care to explore the factors that inhibited or facilitated teamworking in this context. One key finding was that organisational support (e.g. access to resources, senior manager commitment) played an important role in team function. Specifically, they reported that organisational support affected teamworking in four main ways. First, team performance could diminish over time if there was a lack of organisational rewards for improvements in working practices. Second, organisational support helped encourage the use of innovation and implementation of change within teams. Third, a high support for team innovation was often linked to improvements in the quality of teamworking. Fourth, a lack of support to implement team changes was found to encourage apathy from some members in relation to their view of the wider organisation.

Organisational support

As Box 4.3 indicates, organisational support is key for the function of interprofessional teams. Indeed, the rise of the 'new public management' has resulted in a shift in the balance of power from the professions to health and social care managers (Ferlie *et al.*, 1996). Given this increase of management influence, and the fact that most health and social care teams are embedded within organisations, support from management is crucial (e.g. Onyett, 2003; Baxter and Markle-Reid, 2009). Such support ensures that teams have the resources (i.e. time and money) to work together in a largely autonomous fashion, making decisions about how they can collectively respond to the needs of patients.

Jelphs and Dickinson (2008) note that interprofessional teams can sometimes encounter difficulties with their host organisations. They stress that team members will often identify themselves as members of their team, over and above, any connection to the wider organisation in which the team functions. Clearly, this lack of connection can cause a number of challenges, especially when asking for additional funding for recruitment purposes to meet, for example, an increase in service demand.

Other problems can arise when organisational funding arrangements make collaboration between teams based in different institutions compete for limited funding (Fowler *et al.*, 2000). In addition, Koppel (2003) found that organisational support had a harsher edge. On the basis of interviews with primary care physicians, nurses and health service managers, Koppel noted that the physicians and nurses were concerned about an increased organisational control by management in directing their continuing professional development opportunities towards the adoption of team-building activities. As a result of this management influence, the professionals in this study felt their traditional professional autonomy was being eroded (also see Box 5.6).

Professional representation

There are two key forms of professional representation which can affect interprofessional teamwork: representation from professional associations and from unions. Associations representing the range of different health and social care professions, through their policy documents, have been collectively calling for a more interprofessional approach to the delivery of care (see Chapter 2). Along with government support and funding, these professional associations have played a key role in promoting teamwork. However, their policy documents, fail to clearly outline how local health and social care organisations can actually implement or evaluate any of their teamwork activities.

Unions provide health and social care employers with a central bargaining agent and employees (e.g. nurses, therapists) with protection in the workplace. Under the auspices of this relationship, unions, employers and employees can, in principle, create a workplace which is free of discrimination and harassment. Unions can also help professionals feel empowered to report disruptive behaviour, including poor behaviour from their colleagues without concern of retaliation (e.g. Ontario Nurses Association, 2009).

Fear of litigation

The fear of litigation due to an individual error or negligence has been a growing trend in health and social care during the past decade or so. In the US, in particular, practitioners – especially physicians – have reported increasing levels of dissatisfaction and insecurity with their clinical practice generated by fear of litigation (Zuger, 2004). Writing from an interprofessional mental health team perspective, Packman *et al.* (2004) note that while patient suicide is the most feared outcome, 'fear of litigation and liability [. . .] may be a close second' (p. 697). In addition, a fear of possible litigation can provoke secrecy among professions, which can undermine attempts to ensure patient safety. As Berwick (2002, p. 87) notes:

> A culture of safety must be one of openness, honesty, and disclosure, but how is that feasible with a hovering threat of malpractice litigation?

Drawing upon their experiences in New Zealand, where an administrative system of compensation operates without the need to prove fault, Davis *et al.* (2003) noted that professionals tended to work in a more open manner. Their review of patients' hospital records found that the level of acknowledgement of injury in patients' records was remarkably high, which they saw as a consequence of the no fault jurisdiction. In many respects, the recent focus on patient safety, where responsibility for error is widened to include all team members (as well as the organisations in which they work), can be regarded as a response to this fear of individualised litigation.

Contextual factors

Figure 4.1 presented five contextual factors: culture, diversity, gender, economics and politics. Box 4.4 provides an example of how contextual factors, in this case a uniprofessional culture, undermined the quality of teamwork across a number of community mental health teams in the UK.

Culture

The notion of culture is diffuse. Culture may refer to behaviours, beliefs, values, customs as well as institutions. The term can be applied at a societal, organisational or team level. At the societal level, it is possible to identify a wide range of different cultures, often defined by country, region or continent. At the organisational level, a culture has been defined as:

> A patterned system of perceptions, meanings, and beliefs about the organisation which facilitates sense-making amongst a group of people sharing common experiences and guides individual behaviour at work. (Bloor and Dawson, 1994, p. 276)

> **Box 4.4**   An insight into how contextual factors can affect teamwork.
>
> Norman and Peck (1999) report an evaluation of a number of workshops in which community mental health team members (nurses, occupational therapists, social workers and physicians) were asked to generate accounts of their team roles and identities. They found a number of areas in which team members felt they were working well together. These included a strong commitment to teamwork among members; a good shared understanding of each other's roles, methods of working and professional cultures; direct and regular contact between team members; and good communication systems which had led to a high level of trust between the teams and their clients. In addition, the authors identified a range of factors that challenged teamwork, which were linked to an underpinning *uniprofessional culture*. Evidence of this uniprofessional culture were identified as ambiguous professional roles and responsibilities between some members; a lack of agreement around how team members work together in a cooperative fashion; differences in professional power, status and income between members; the existence of conflicting caseload priorities within the teams; and the use of different models of care between members, which generated different objectives and working methods.

At the team level, culture can similarly be seen as the meanings and perceptions different team members attach to their team as well as their interprofessional interactions.

Because meaning is constructed between the individuals who work within teams and organisations, attaining shared agreement is an ongoing process. As a result, while team and organisational members may share some meanings, they are open to wide range of interpretations (e.g. Morgan, 1986). Understanding organisational culture involves an exploration of power relations to explain how individuals and groups create and contest meaning and how they use the resources to which they have access, including interprofessional teams, to advance their particular viewpoints and agendas (e.g. Wright, 1994; Albert *et al.*, 2009).

Sociological studies by authors such as Becker *et al.* (1961) and Melia (1987) have provided rich insights into the nature of the professional cultures of medicine and nursing. Their work has revealed how professionals develop distinctive and contrasting cultures that encompass a range of particular values, beliefs, attitudes, customs and behaviours which, as we discussed above, are effectively transferred from one generation to the next through a process of professional socialisation. Drawing upon such work, Hall (2005) noted that these professional cultures evolved as the different professions developed, reflecting historic as well as social and gender factors. Educational and professional experiences that occur reinforce the common values, approaches and language of each profession. Specialisation within professions, she argued, has led to even further immersion into the knowledge and culture of these speciality groups. As a result, Hall regarded professional cultures as a central factor which can impede the development of interprofessional teamwork.

At a micro level, interprofessional teams also create their own particular local cultures, which help shape how members interact and work together. For example, in their study of interprofessional relationships between two teams based in a geriatric assessment unit, Gair and Hartery (2001) revealed a team culture which centred on medical, nursing, physiotherapy and occupational therapy input into team decisions, but often excluded input from other members such as health visitors, social workers and speech therapists.

Diversity

We live in a diverse world in which different cultures, social, political and economic systems, organisations and professions coexist. Like culture, diversity operates at societal, organisational and team levels. Health and social care teams are diverse – they emerge for different reasons, function in many different ways across a variety of settings (Meerabeau and Page, 1999).

Diversity within teams can have a number of benefits, including an enhanced expertise and experience from which to draw upon in their work (Handy, 1999). Indeed, organisational studies have suggested that diverse teams can collaborate in more innovative ways due to their depth of collective knowledge than more homogenous teams (e.g. Kochan *et al.*, 2003).

Despite the value placed on diversity, Firth-Cozens (2001) has argued that 'the reality is that working together from a variety of perspectives is sometimes difficult to achieve' (p. 65). Moreover, the diversity generated by professional socialisation and the professionalisation processes has resulted in the emergence of a diversity of views and cultures. It has also generated inequality of economic rewards, social status and professional power, which as discussed above, can be problematic for interprofessional teamwork.

Gender

Gender inequalities in the form of patriarchy – an arrangement in which men occupy dominant social, economic and political positions across society (Witz, 1992) – is a key element that shapes the nature of interprofessional relationships within health and social care (e.g. Davies, 1995; Porter, 1995; Wickes, 1998).

In her analysis of the development of nursing (in relation to medicine), Gamarnikow (1978) argued that the profession followed paternal relations of the Victorian family in the world of work, whereby medicine made up largely of men, assumed the role as the head of the household, and women, assumed the more subordinate, supportive roles. As most other professions (e.g. occupational therapy, dietetics, speech and language therapy) are composed largely of women, arguably, this has resulted in similar patriarchal relations with medicine. Interprofessional team relations between these professions therefore can be seen to reproduce the traditional patriarchal arrangements.

Medicine is, however, becoming more feminised. In the last few years the number of female medical students has exceeded 50% in many western countries (Levinson and Lurie, 2004). Given this evolving picture within medicine, the patriarchal nature of interprofessional health and social care relations will also shift. At present though, it is difficult to predict the nature of this shift, and how it may affect the other inequalities which exist between medicine and the other professions.

Political will

Political will, in the form of policies advocating interprofessional teamwork, has played a significant role in promoting teamwork around the globe (see Chapter 2). Over the past decade one can see political willingness for teamwork from the national governments of a number of countries such as the UK, the US and Australia, as well as from a range of regional governments in these and other countries. Collectively, this political will has helped create a climate for teamwork and released funds to support the development and implementation of a range of teamwork initiatives (see Box 2.3). Political will can also elicit commitment from professional bodies (e.g. the UK Nursing and Midwifery Council and the Association of American Medical Colleges) and can foster the development of initiatives such as patient safety and their supporting agencies (e.g. the UK National Patient Safety Agency and the Australian Patient Safety Foundation) which demand effective interprofessional teamwork to reduce error.

While political will from a variety of international, national and regional governments, and professional associations has been a crucial element in the development of interprofessional teamwork, their supporting policy documents are often problematic. For example, as noted above, they provide little direction or guidance about the development or delivery of teamwork activities, leaving complex implementation tasks up to locally based organisations. In addition, these documents fail to pay attention to key underlying factors in teamwork (e.g. power and status imbalances), which, as we have discussed in this chapter, play a critical role in shaping the nature of interprofessional relations in teams.

Economics

Despite very plausible arguments about teamwork helping to achieve economic gains (e.g. improved communication between team members reduces duplication of effort and resource wastage), there is little evidence on cost-effectiveness for interprofessional teamwork across health and social care settings. Although, as Oxman et al. (2008) note, economic factors can play a significant role in affecting the delivery of integrated team-based care. For instance, the introduction of financial incentives such as pay-for-performance can result in interprofessional teams 'cherry-picking' patients where good outcomes can be achieved over those where such outcomes are more difficult to realise.

Given the differences in influence and status achieved by the different professionalisation processes, each of the professions has achieved different levels of economic rewards, with physicians being able to achieve higher incomes than their colleagues. Unlike Europe, where most health care professionals are paid a salary, in North America, physicians' remuneration is still based on a 'pay-for-service' model. This has resulted in them being able to command significantly higher incomes than their salaried colleagues. Indeed, the way in which the financial reward is provided may lead to conflicts in objectives between professionals (e.g. Wertheimer *et al.*, 2008). For example, nurses who are public-sector-salaried employees may seek out low stress, high quality and collaborative care while self-employed fee-for-service physicians may prioritise effective technical decisions with little engagement in activities which are not reimbursed.

Conclusions and implications

Individually and collectively, the factors discussed in this chapter can have a significant effect on the performance of interprofessional teams. For example, hierarchical differences between team members place them in different social and economic relations with one another. This can undermine the quality of their relations. In addition, the roles which members adopt can either generate friction (if roles are unclear) or support team performance (if roles are negotiated and agreed between members). The processual factors presented indicate how the nature of elements such as time and space, routines and rituals, and unpredictability can affect how interprofessional teamwork is actually undertaken. For example, limited time and too many demands can mean professionals have little opportunity to focus on strengthening their collaborative work. As we discussed, organisational factors including support for resources of time and money are key to the effective functioning of interprofessional teams. The focus related to the contextual factors presented above adds width to the issues surrounding teamwork. For example, differences in financial rewards may emphasise different values among different members of the team.

Our aim in developing and presenting our framework has been to convey the complexity of interprofessional teamwork from a range of different standpoints: relational, processual, organisational and contextual. While we presented the factors separately, they are interconnected in a number of ways. We describe later how, for example, they could be interwoven into interventions to improve teamworking and ensure that it has a firm conceptual underpinning.

5 Using theory to better understand interprofessional teamwork

Introduction

Accounts of interprofessional teamwork rarely draw upon theory. For example, while imbalances of power are often mentioned in studies of teamworking, theory is seldom used to provide deeper insights. In this chapter we draw together a number of social science theories from psychodynamics, systems, social psychology, sociology and organisational sources. We frame this discussion using our four teamwork factors – relational, processual, organisation and contextual – to show how different theories can yield different insights and understandings of interprofessional teamwork. For readers who have only a limited knowledge of the role of social science theory, we initially provide an outline of its nature and how we have used social science perspectives to inform our own work. We then present, discuss and critique a range of pertinent social science theories in order to provide a better understanding of the complexities of interprofessional teamwork. For each of those that we discuss, we illustrate how the theory has been applied to a study of interprofessional teamwork.

Understanding the nature of theory

Social science theories provide complex and comprehensive understandings of phenomena that are not easily explained, such as how societies work, how organisations operate and why people interact in certain ways. Theory provides different 'lenses' through which to look at complicated problems and social issues, focusing on different aspects of a phenomenon and providing a framework for understanding them. Theories also generate knowledge that can be generalised across settings.

Merton (1968) outlined three types of theory:

- Grand or macro theory – which is non-specific and constructed from relatively abstract concepts that are difficult to operationalise and empirically test.
- Mid-range theory – which is more limited in scope, as it addresses specific phenomena and has a limited number of concepts relating to a restricted range of contexts.
- Micro or practice theory – which has the narrowest range of interest, as it is focused on specific phenomena and contexts.

Theories can be generated explicitly from data or developed implicitly from personal constructions about particular phenomena. Data-driven theories are easier to implement in practice, as their development is usually recorded and therefore easier to follow. Implicit theories (sometimes termed 'armchair' or 'guru' theories) are different as they are more:

> Akin to an experienced cook who knows the basic components, how they interact, and how many pinches or handfuls of ingredients are required to produce the desired product. (ICEBeRG, 2006, p. 4)

As a result, such theories are more difficult to implement in practice.

For those interested in reading more about the nature, role and contribution of social science theory see, for example, Crotty (1998).

Using a social science lens

As we noted previously, we have adopted a *social science* approach to seeing the world – a standpoint which we use in this book to explore and understand the nature of interprofessional teamwork. In offering this particular perspective we are mindful of Wright Mills (1959) who, just over 50 years ago, argued for the need to employ a social science lens to view the world and understand the nature of people's actions and interactions. He went on to note that as, 'neither the life of an individual nor the history of a society can be understood without understanding both' (p. 3), exploration of the links between individuals and their societies was critical. For Wright Mills, developing of an understanding of the social world requires connecting research with social science theory. Without making connections between theory and research, he argued, such accounts offer nothing more than *abstracted empiricism*. Social science perspectives are therefore needed to generate more comprehensive and meaningful accounts of the nature of the social world.

Theories in this chapter

We have selected a number of different social science theories to help us comprehend the intricacies of teamworking in health and social care – these theories are listed in Table 5.1.

Table 5.1 Social science theories that aid better understanding of interprofessional teamwork.

Factor	Theoretical approach	Type	Teamwork focus
Relational	Psychodynamic perspectives (Bion, Menzies, Marris)	Micro	Unconscious processes related to team function
	Social psychological perspectives (Tajfel and Turner, Brown)	Micro	Social identity and conflict
	Interactionism (Goffman, Strauss)	Micro	Team interactions
Processual	Activity theory (Engeström)	Mid-range	Completion of team tasks and activities
Organisational	Institutional influence (DiMaggio and Powell)	Mid-range	Influence of institutions on team relations and team performance
Contextual	Professionalisation (Freidson)	Mid-range	Closure between professions
	Discourse theory (Foucault)	Grand	Wider influences of social power on interprofessional teamwork
	Surveillance theory (Foucault)	Grand	

While we recognise that there are a vast number of other social science theories that could be selected, we have chosen those above for three main reasons:

- They help to illuminate all of the different elements – relational, processual, organisational and contextual – of our conceptual framework
- They offer different micro-level (e.g. Goffman), mid-range (e.g. Freidson) and grand theory (e.g. Foucault) perspectives, thus providing a diversity of ideas that can be applied to multiple phenomena
- They were developed, in part, from studies within the context of health care and/or are applied widely in health and social care.

For some, the inclusion of a range of different theoretical approaches, each with its own distinct epistemological roots, might be considered simply providing a 'theory soup'. However, it is useful to remember that a number of seemingly contrasting theoretical approaches can have more in common than one may initially suspect. For example, Hacking (2004) argues that despite apparent theoretical differences, Goffman's and Foucault's perspectives are complementary. The former focuses on understanding how people interact within an existing institution while the latter provides ways in which to understand how individuals' interactions are shaped by the culture (e.g. norms, behaviours and language) they live and work within. Both approaches are therefore useful for understanding the nature of interaction *and* the nature of the surrounding institutions in which interactions occur. Furthermore, our pluralistic stance encourages us to embrace a range of contrasting theoretical contributions as this can provide more comprehensive insights into the nature of a particular phenomenon.

Relational perspectives

In this section we draw on social theories from three different traditions – psychodynamics, social psychology and sociology – that help understand relational perspectives.

Unconscious processes in teams

We discuss the psychodynamic work of Wilfred Bion, Isabel Menzies and Peter Marris, which aims to theorise about the role that unconscious processes can play in interprofessional teamwork.

Early work by Bion (1961) on work-group mentality theory attempts to explain the unconscious processes involved in groups and teams unable to manage their (collective and consciously agreed) 'primary task'. According to Bion, groups will often waste time and avoid making decisions in order to prevent members from tackling potentially difficult group issues which arise in the completion of their primary task. Bion's work was later applied to hospital teams by Menzies (1970) in the development of her theory of social defence. For Menzies, members of hospital teams have two tasks: the primary one of patient care and a secondary one of maintaining the team (e.g. managing team relations). Menzies noted that under stressful circumstances, and in certain teams with poor clarity of goals and leadership, the secondary task can replace the primary one as a mechanism of dealing with the stress. For example, individuals who normally collaborate well with other professions to deliver care can become defensive during times of anxiety (for example due to staff shortages), and find it difficult to achieve the primary task of delivering care. One coping mechanism for dealing with this anxiety might be to withdraw from their collaborative work. Menzies also noted that the following psychodynamic processes could emerge in teams:

- Denial – where individuals continue to reject viewpoints or arguments despite overwhelming evidence
- Splitting – the separation of 'good' or gratifying objects or actions from 'bad' or frustrating ones
- Projection – where individuals' personal attributes, thoughts or emotions are ascribed onto others.

More recently, Marris (1986) developed a theory centred upon loss and change which suggests that individuals often experience emotions of loss when change occurs. Marris maintains that fear of such changes may contribute to unconscious feelings of anxiety, which could in turn create resistance to change. Box 5.1 provides an illustration of the use of Marris's work to illuminate the nature of interprofessional collaboration within an older adult care setting in the UK.

> **Box 5.1** The use of Marris's psychodynamic theory on loss and change.
>
> In their study of an interprofessional initiative for staff working together in an older adult care setting, Holman and Jackson (2001) found that unconscious processes between team members played an important role in the way that they worked together. Participants included nurses, a psychologist, a bereavement officer and a chaplain. The initiative focused on bereavement and combined information giving with reflective workshops. Findings from interviews with these participants indicated that their approach to interprofessional collaboration and teamwork was not altered, although they enjoyed their interprofessional experiences. The authors drew on Marris's psychodynamic theory in their analysis to argue that the failure of staff to change their practice after participating in the workshops was due to resistance generated from unconscious feelings of anxiety about possible changes in their interprofessional work practices.

Obholzer and Zagier Roberts (1994) have drawn on the theories developed by Bion and Menzies to provide an analysis of how psychodynamic processes operate across a number of health and social care organisations, and to describe some of the problems (e.g. denial and projection) which can occur between professionals working together in interprofessional teams. Van Der Walt and Swartz (2002) have also used this approach to explain the persistence of task-oriented nursing and the difficulties of instituting change in clinic teams within a tuberculosis control programme in South Africa.

Social identity and conflict

Two related social psychological theories are presented in this section – the work of Tajfel and Turner (1986) on social identity theory and of Brown *et al.* (1986) on realistic conflict theory.

Social identity theory proposes that a person will identify more closely with members from their own social group (e.g. family, profession or organisation) than with members from other groups. The theory was originally developed by Tajfel and Turner (1986) to understand the social psychological basis of intergroup discrimination and the conditions that would lead group members to discriminate in favour of the 'in-group' to which they belonged and against other 'out-groups'. Tajfel and Turner argued that the act of individuals categorising themselves as group members was sufficient to lead them to display in-group favouritism. After being categorised as a group member, individuals would seek to achieve self-esteem by positively differentiating their in-group from a comparison out-group.

A closely related approach is realistic conflict theory (Brown *et al.*, 1986) which assumes that groups holding divergent objectives will have hostile and discriminatory intergroup relations, whereas groups with common objectives will display conciliatory behaviour. Hostility between groups is regarded as a result of direct competition for limited and valued resources. If the outcomes of two groups are competitively interdependent (gains for one group result in losses for the other), intergroup hostility will be maximised. Consequently, negative out-group stereotypes, increased in-group solidarity and cohesiveness will be emphasised. If the groups are cooperatively interdependent (e.g. there are shared goals), intergroup hostility will be reduced, cumulatively improving intergroup relations.

These theories have been used widely in the interprofessional literature to help explore the nature of tensions which can arise when two or more professionals come together in a practice or educational setting (e.g. Carpenter and Hewstone, 1996; Hind *et al.*, 2003; Pollard *et al.*, 2006). Box 5.2 provides an example of the application of social identity theory.

Box 5.2   The use of Tajfel and Turner's social identity theory.

Mandy *et al.* (2004) employed social identity theory to help understand the findings of a study that evaluated the impact of an interprofessional education programme delivered to physiotherapy and podiatry students. The programme's aim was to provide learners from these two professions with an opportunity to understand and value their respective roles within an interprofessional health and social care context. Survey findings indicated that students' initial negative stereotypes of one another's professions were reinforced following the delivery of the course. In discussing their findings, Mandy and colleagues argued that the limited effect of this interprofessional experience can be usefully understood by drawing upon social identity theory. They note that, 'the different professions each have their own distinct occupational culture, which will lead to distinct tribal groups. Each professional group will develop its own characteristic style of communication and language, which in turn leads to stereotypical judgements' (Mandy *et al.*, 2004, p. 165). In employing social identity theory, the authors argue that negative stereotypes are difficult to change, given the nature of intergroup discrimination.

In addition, Hean *et al.* (2006) have employed social identity theory to explore the effects of early professional socialisation processes of health and social care students. Overall, they found that students from a number of professions, including midwifery, medicine, nursing, occupational therapy, pharmacy and physiotherapy perceived their in-group identities as being very distinct from other professional groups.

Team interactions

The work of two sociologists is presented in this section – Anselm Strauss's negotiated order perspective and Erving Goffman's theory of impression management.

Strauss *et al.*'s (1963) negotiated order perspective was developed in reaction to earlier explanations of social order within organisations. These tended to stress formal structures and rules, and neglect the influence of micro-level negotiations. On the basis of research in a psychiatric hospital, Strauss and colleagues proposed that professionals, patients and lay workers negotiate meanings, routines and work. These negotiations took place within the context of the formal goals and methods of how psychiatric care *ought* to be delivered. Indeed, through these data Strauss and colleagues came to view interaction and negotiation as a core aspect of organisational life. In particular, they found that negotiation between individuals (e.g. bargaining, compromising and mediating) around formal rules and structures essentially shaped the nature of organisational life. As a result, they argued, these micro-level negotiations contributed to the maintenance of the 'social order' which exists within each organisation.

Strauss (1978) later modified this theory to address concerns that it failed to pay sufficient attention to the influence of structural factors. He subsequently suggested that although micro-level negotiation was central to creating and maintaining organisational life, negotiations were constrained by the existence of structural influences. However, Strauss continued to argue that while macro influences provided the parameters for relationships, micro-level negotiations still played a key role in forming and shaping organisational life.

Strauss's negotiated order perspective has been used widely to understand how micro-level negotiations shape organisations (e.g. Busch, 1982). For example, Cott (1998) employed this approach to explore and understand the nature of hierarchy and interprofessional teamwork within a rehabilitation setting (see Box 4.1). In addition, Svensson (1996) used the theory to explore the nature of nurse–doctor negotiations regarding decisions on patient care.

We move on now to consider Erving Goffman's theory of impression management. Goffman (1963) developed his theory from anthropological fieldwork exploring the nature of social interactions. He found that communication between individuals took the form of linguistic (verbal) and non-linguistic (body language) gestures employed when individuals presented their selves to others. He revealed that individuals over-communicate gestures that reinforce their desired self and under-communicate gestures that detract from this self perception. He termed this process 'impression management'.

For Goffman, the presentation process was seen as a 'performance', which was undertaken in two distinct areas: public 'front region performances', such as meetings between work colleagues or professional–patient consultations; and private 'back region performances', such as interactions between friends and family members. He argued that front region performances were generally formal and restrained in nature, in contrast to back region performances which were more informal, allowing the individual to 'relax [...] and step out of [their front region] character' (Goffman, 1963, p. 115). Importantly, Goffman viewed backstage regions as key locations where individuals could prepare for their front stage performances. He therefore regarded the activities that took place in private settings as crucial to supporting the activities that occurred in public settings. Each region, then, is seen to have different 'rules' of behaviour that shape the ways in which individuals present themselves.

Goffman's theory has been drawn on widely to explain 'performances' within health care. For example, research on medical and nursing students has indicated the significance of front and backstage performances, and how the backstage is employed to help prepare for front stage performance during their professional socialisation (Broadhead, 1983; Melia, 1987). Ellingson (2005) also employed Goffman's theory in her study of team interactions within a geriatric oncology setting in the US (see Box 5.3).

Box 5.3   The use of a sociological perspective – Goffman's interactionist approach.

Ellingson's work exploring the nature of backstage informal interprofessional communication revealed that this form of communication played a central role in progressing patient care. Professionals, she found, had fewer interruptions and could speak more candidly about patient care issues in the backstage than in the front stage locations of the clinic. In total, she identified seven types of communication which used front and backstage settings, ranging from informal (backstage) information sharing to more formal (front stage) communications such as written reports. Ellingson's study also indicated that there was a certain degree of fluidity between backstage and front stage areas within the clinic. For example, the opening of a meeting room door could instantly reveal interprofessional backstage communication to the scrutiny of others looking in from outside.

More recently, one of us (Reeves, 2008) drew upon Goffman's work to explore the uses of formal and informal performances within an interprofessional planning group established to develop and implement an interprofessional initiative for students from four professional groups.

Processual perspectives

Processual factors focus on understanding how the interprofessional work processes undertaken by a team may be affected by issues such as time, space and task complexity. Given this focus, we have drawn upon an approach which illuminates the nature of *how* work is undertaken in organisations – activity theory.

Activity theory

Activity theory was originally rooted in the work of Vygotsky (1978) and later developed by Engeström *et al.* (1999). It helps to explain how social interactions and relations are affected by different forms of activities. As such, it includes a focus on the full range of 'activity systems' which exist within social encounters. Activity systems, Engeström and colleagues stated, replicate the nature of the multifaceted communication that occurs between humans, within the social and physical structures involved in their work. Activity systems consist of the following elements: individuals, objectives, tools, communities and rules. Knotworking is a key concept within this theory. Its use can help understand how, for example, interprofessional teamwork is undertaken through a combination of professionals coming from their own specific activity systems and bringing with them their own threads of activity. These separate threads of activities are tied, untied and retied during their work together to provide care. These multiple threads are described as a 'knotworking knot'. In interprofessional teams, knots are continuously modified depending upon the nature of the activity and the interacting individuals. Box 5.4 provides an example of how two of us employed this theory to understand the nature of interprofessional collaboration within general medical wards.

Box 5.4   The use of Engeström's activity theory in medical wards.

Our study, based in a general and emergency medical directorate of a large inner city teaching hospital in the UK, examined the meanings that different professionals attached to their interprofessional work (Reeves and Lewin, 2004). Data gathered included interviews with doctors, nurses, therapists and social workers, and participant observation of ward-based work. We found that interprofessional collaboration consisted largely of short, unstructured and often opportunistic interactions. We also found the wards to be busy and therefore not conducive to drawn out discussions. On these words, a large number of professionals entered and left during a single day – up to 15 doctors from five or six different medical teams, ten members of the nursing staff, three to four therapists, two social workers, a pharmacist, and two care coordinators. In this context, the notion of a clearly defined interprofessional team was misleading. Rather, interprofessional interactions were more loosely formed and transient in nature, largely suggestive of the concept of knotworking in which professionals came together to tie and untie interactive threads of activity in their work.

Activity theory has also been employed by others including Freeth *et al.* (2006) in their work describing an interprofessional session delivered to different professionals working within a maternity setting who formed 'teams' for a one-day simulation activity. Varpio *et al.* (2008) also draw on this theory in their work on interprofessional communication and medical error in acute care settings.

Organisational perspectives

Organisational factors are concerned with exploring the local environment in which the interprofessional team operates and how organisational structures and processes affect the interprofessional team. The theory of institutional influence is drawn upon to understand these issues.

The influence of the institution

DiMaggio and Powell (1983) developed their theory based on Weber's early sociological work which viewed the increasing rationalisation of social life as an 'iron cage' of rule-based rational control. They emphasise the role of institutional control, arguing that organisations have a tendency to preserve and enhance their own legitimation.

DiMaggio and Powell suggest that there are three key processes which affect organisational legitimation: 'coercive' forces or pressures exerted on the organisation from external sources such as regulatory agencies; 'mimetic' forces which result in organisations imitating their peers as a way of dealing with uncertainty; and 'normative' forces linked to the professionals who work within the organisations. They argue that the collective outcome of these forces is for organisations to function in a state of 'isomorphism' – where they resemble one another.

Within health and social care, organisations are becoming increasingly isomorphic in nature due to pressures from government policy and regulatory agencies to reorganise themselves to provide more team-based care. While DiMaggio and Powell's approach has not been applied widely in health and social care contexts, there are a few useful examples. Russell (1990) employed the approach in an analysis of the functioning of hospice programmes. This study showed that, in general, hospices operated in an isomorphic fashion and tended to be characterised by processes which counteracted change and thus maintained the status quo. More recently, Ginsburg and Tregunno (2005) employed institutional theory to understand how interprofessional education and collaboration may be coercive forces in the context of organisational change within health care.

Contextual perspectives

Contextual factors consider the broad cultural, political, social and economic landscape in which the team is located. Theories developed by Friedson and Foucault help to understand the effects of these wider phenomena on teamwork.

Professionalisation

Sociologically, work by Freidson (1970) offered a critical turning point in thinking about professions, as traditional accounts tended to stress their functionality, universalism and neutrality. Based on his exploration of the development of medicine, Freidson argued that occupational groups actively engage in a process of professionalisation through engagement of 'closure'. The aim of this process was straightforward – to secure exclusive ownership of specific areas of knowledge and expertise in order to effectively secure economic reward and status enhancement.

Another key part of the professionalisation of occupational groups was the licensing of their practice through their connections with the state. Without this formal link, granting the right to a monopoly of practice, it was argued that an occupation cannot successfully achieve professional closure. As Larkin (1983, p. 48) stated:

> A profession's relationship with the state [...] is fundamental. Occupations that attempt to secure for themselves the two dimensions of professionalism – market control and social mobility – generally seek to establish a legal monopoly through licensure by the state.

Freidson claimed that in order to protect the gains obtained from professionalisation, all occupational groups guard the areas of knowledge and expertise that they have acquired. This is done primarily through the regulation of entry and the maintenance of professional standards. Tension is therefore likely to arise if it is perceived that a member from another profession is infringing their area of expertise. Reflecting upon this feature of professionalisation, Abbott (1988, p. 2) stated:

> A fundamental fact of professional life [is] interprofessional competition. It is the history of [this competition] that is the real, determining history of professions.

One can see similarities in how each of the health and social care occupations has engaged in their respective professionalisation processes. However, as medicine was the first to successfully professionalise, it has been argued that it claimed the most prestigious areas of clinical work – the ability to diagnose and prescribe (e.g. Macdonald, 1995). Over the years, despite the introduction of new roles such as the nurse practitioner, which have made advances into medicine's clinical domain, it has been argued that medicine has largely maintained its status (e.g. Witz, 1992; Porter, 1995). Nevertheless, through both the timing of their professionalisation process and prestigious nature of the areas of knowledge and expertise medicine claimed, in relation to the other professions, one can see that a clear hierarchy operates within the health and social care professions. Medicine occupies the dominant position in this hierarchy based on the gains from its professionalisation process. Box 5.5 provides an example of contemporary professional boundary protectionism in the area of sports medicine.

Box 5.5   The use the professionalisation approach to understand medical sports teams.

Theberge (2008) examined the integration of chiropractors into interprofessional teams in the area of sports medicine. The study was based on interviews with 35 health professionals, including physicians, physiotherapists, athletic therapists and chiropractors. Findings from this study supported the notion that 'athletes wanted them', which helped chiropractors secure a position within the system of sports medicine professionals. Yet their position was marked by ongoing tensions with other professions (e.g. medicine and physiotherapy) over their scope and content of practice. Chiropractors' success in achieving acceptance within sports medicine teams was, it appeared, contingent on a reduced scope of practice in which they offered only a limited range of treatments.

This theoretical approach has also been usefully employed to understand why friction can occur during interprofessional education activities (e.g. Connolly, 1995) as well as to explore professional boundary maintenance between health care staff working in cardiac care (e.g. Sanders and Harrison, 2008).

Discourse and surveillance

According to Foucault (1972), a discourse helps to define a particular culture, its language and the behaviour of individuals who belong to that culture. Discourses are knowledge systems of ideas, attitudes, actions, beliefs and practices that influence how individuals think, see and speak. Discourses therefore have the power to shape a culture and define what becomes accepted as 'truth' and 'fact'. For Foucault, discourses are also key in legitimating the position of the powerful – those who create and shape the discourses which generate what is regarded as the truth.

While discourses shape culture and language, Foucault (1979) believed that surveillance was required to help maintain the existence of a particular discourse. Therefore, Foucault saw surveillance as another dimension of power. Foucault drew upon the notion of the *panopticon* – a prison building designed by Jeremy Bentham, in which prisoners were not aware of when they were being watched by guards, thereby inducing acts of self-surveillance and providing the guards with psychological power over the inmates. Foucault used this idea to illustrate the powerful nature of surveillance in a wider social context. Indeed, for Foucault, the use of surveillance and self-surveillance were crucial forms of power that ensured individuals remained compliant to a particular discourse. Box 5.6 provides an example of how these perspectives have been applied to an interprofessional setting.

Other work on interprofessional teams has also drawn upon Foucault's theories. For example, Regan de Bere (2003) employed discourse theory to explore how mental health teams could generate a 'shared team discourse' as a result of team training activities. In addition, Opie (2001) employed theories of discourse and surveillance in her work on the nature of power imbalances between different professions working in health and social care teams.

Implications for teamwork

Individually, the theories presented in this chapter offer a range of valuable insights for interprofessional teamwork. The psychodynamic theories of Bion (1961), Menzies (1970) and Marris (1986) highlight how underlying unconscious processes may affect the ways individuals work together in an interprofessional team. The ambivalent and intertwined histories of the professions, as well as the complexities of organising care, may all conspire to overwhelm the primary task of such teams. In addition, the social psychological theories of Tajfel and Turner (1986) and Brown *et al.* (1986) offer insights into how individuals identify with

---

Box 5.6 The use of Foucauldian theory in primary care teams.

Koppel (2003) explored how the growing influence of health service management affected the education of health care professionals based in primary care teams. Drawing on interviews with physicians, nurses and health service managers, he reported that these professionals were particularly concerned about the increased control that managers had over their continuing professional development activities. Consequently, they felt that management was attempting to control their behaviour and erode their autonomy. Employing Foucault's theories of discourse and surveillance, Koppel argued that, supported by government policy, management had employed a 'discourse of efficiency' to advocate the use of interprofessional education to ensure that professionals would learn and then work together in a more 'efficient' manner. For Koppel, surveillance within interprofessional education was a central element in controlling professional behaviour. By learning together, individuals were open to scrutiny from other professions. Thus, a profession's uniqueness of knowledge and expertise could be questioned, as each was open to a critique of their actions, thoughts and attitudes. Consequently, their autonomy was undermined and 'moulded' to fit into the management-led discourse.

---

certain professions, teams and organisations (in-groups) and how this may, in turn, create tensions for teamwork with others (out-groups) who do not have this membership and are therefore considered 'outsiders'.

The use of activity theory (Engeström *et al.*, 1999) may help to understand how interprofessional interactions and team relations are affected by the activities that team members undertake. The knotworking concept has already begun to be employed to explore how collaboration, under pressure, may shift from teamworking towards knotworking. The theory of institutional influence developed by DiMaggio and Powell (1983) offers further insights into the interplay between organisations and the professionals who work within them. It also helps understand the 'forces' which result in many organisations having similar structures, policies and personnel. The use of this theory may inform ideas about how interprofessional teamwork acts as a 'coercive' force on organisational function.

The sociological theories of Strauss (1978) and Goffman (1963), and of Freidson (1970) and Foucault (1972, 1979) help understand the nature of interprofessional teamwork from three vantage points. Strauss's and Goffman's work offers micro-level insights into how individuals negotiate and interact across different social and clinical settings. By contrast, Freidson's work provides a macro-level understanding of how occupational closure processes generate boundaries which professions then maintain and protect. Foucault's work offers a broader view of the social processes which underpin interprofessional teamwork. It highlights the role of power in constructing different discourses (including a teamwork discourse), as well as how surveillance can be used by those in dominant positions as a way of monitoring and influencing those in more subordinate positions.

Collectively, these theoretical approaches help enhance our understanding of interprofessional teamwork. They cover the foci of our four teamwork factors (relational, processual, organisational and contextual); they represent a range of disciplinary traditions (psychodynamics, systems, social psychology, sociology and organisational studies) and provide a variety of theoretical standpoints (micro, mid-range and grand theory).

Limitations of the theories

While these perspectives help to understand the nature of interprofessional teamwork, and provide a basis for considering how one might intervene to improve teamwork, they nevertheless have a number of limitations.

The focus of psychodynamic theories (such as those of Bion, Menzies and Marris) on unconscious processes means that generating convincing evidence to link these processes to interprofessional teamwork actions is extremely difficult. Of the sociological theories that we have discussed, Freidson's theory of professionalisation can be criticised for its singular focus on the macro-level process of closure which overlooks individual resistance. Similarly, the focus of both Strauss's and Goffman's work on individual interactions can be critiqued for failing to take into account the broader social processes (which Freidson's theory aims to uncover).

The social psychological theories of Tajfel and Turner, and also of Brown and colleagues, can be criticised for an over emphasis on small, group-based processes at the expense of wider social and contextual factors, such as gender and culture. The organisational work of DiMaggio and Powell may be critiqued for not giving sufficient attention to the impact individual interactions can have on organisational function. Similarly, both activity theory and Foucault's work may be criticised for their macro-level (or grand theory) focus which may overlook the role of individuals and their micro-level interactions.

Conclusions

In this chapter we have drawn together a range of social science theories that help to deepen our understanding of interprofessional teamwork. Their use can also be extremely beneficial to the development and evaluation of teamwork interventions. We framed the discussion in this chapter using our four teamwork factors – relational, processual, organisational and contextual – to show how different theories can yield differing insights and understandings of interprofessional teamwork. These theories were selected because they were developed within the context of health care, draw on a number of social science disciplines and provide different (micro, mid-range and macro) levels of explanation of social phenomena such as teamworking.

6 Interprofessional teamwork interventions

Introduction

In this chapter we explore the use of different interventions designed to enhance interprofessional teamwork. We define an interprofessional intervention as a consciously developed and implemented activity which aims to change the ways in which interprofessional teams work together, often with the primary purpose of improving quality or efficiency of care provision. We initially discuss work which aims to improve the conceptual clarity of interprofessional interventions. We then review a range of teamwork interventions which we have organised according to each of the four domains – contextual, relational, processual and organisational – of the framework discussed in Chapter 4.

Classifying interprofessional interventions

Despite a growing amount of research on interprofessional interventions to promote collaboration and teamwork, a systematic review that two of us undertook indicated a continuing problem with the conceptualisation of different types of interprofessional *educational* and *practice* interventions (Zwarenstein and Reeves, 2006). Clarity has been inhibited by the lack of a robust evidence base for the effects of these interventions, resulting in confusion between them, as can be seen in the variety of overlapping terms employed, such as 'interprofessional learning', 'interdisciplinary teamwork' and 'transdisciplinary practice'. Leathard (1994, p. 5) originally termed this problem a 'terminological quagmire' – a situation which was relatively unchanged when she revisited the field nearly a decade later (Leathard, 2003a).

Funded by a recent Canadian Institutes of Health Research grant, and working with research, educational, clinical and policymaking colleagues, we conducted a scoping review to develop an empirically tested understanding of interprofessional interventions (including teamwork). This project has involved developing a model to help categorise interprofessional interventions. Findings from an analysis of over 100 papers revealed three main types of interprofessional intervention:

- *Education-based interventions*: Defined as those which included a curriculum with explicitly stated learning objectives/outcomes and learning activities (e.g. teamwork exercises, simulation, site visits and placements). Examples ranged from pre-qualification interprofessional education initiatives, which aimed to develop teamwork skills, to post-qualification interprofessional education activities, which focused on developing knowledge of different team members' professional roles.
- *Practice-based interventions*: Defined as those which aimed to improve how professionals interact in practice. Examples included the use of interprofessional meetings as well as communication tools such as checklists.
- *Organisation-based interventions*: Defined as those which aimed to affect interprofessional collaboration or teamwork by the use of organisational means. This included the introduction of staffing policies or guidelines designed to enhance teamwork or the reconfiguration of workspace to promote the frequency and quality of interprofessional interactions.

While many of the studies included in our scoping review employed a single intervention (typically educational), some did use a multifaceted approach. These included, for example, an educational *and* a practice-based intervention. However, studies that employed two or more interventions often conflated them under the rubric of an 'interprofessional intervention'. We were therefore unable to distinguish between the effects of the education- and practice-based approaches used. Conflation was compounded by a similar failure to tease out different outcomes, as studies typically employed interchangeable and poorly defined terms such as 'teamwork', 'collaboration', 'communication' and 'coordination'.

The overall quality of the evaluations in these studies varied. While we found some of high quality, many of the interprofessional education-based studies were evaluated using only participant perceptions of the initiative in relation to changes in their knowledge and attitudes. In addition, studies that examined teamwork and collaboration used tools such as the Team Climate Inventory (see Appendix 4) or examined the content of team communication. However, neither the processes of teamwork nor their link to health and social care outcomes were investigated. More information on this scoping review can be found in Reeves *et al.* (2009b) and Goldman *et al.* (2009).

We go on to employ this typology to help frame our discussion of the different interprofessional teamwork interventions below.

Teamwork interventions

In this section we present a selection of interventions designed to improve interprofessional teamwork. Building on the discussion of our framework in Chapter 4, we have organised the different interventions using the following four factors: relational, processual, organisational and contextual. As we go on to note, while a number of interventions, such as team training, are examples of 'direct' team-work interventions (i.e. they aim to affect teamwork directly), others such as case management are more 'indirect' in nature. For such 'indirect' interventions, their effects on teamwork form only part of the intervention, which is aimed primarily at improving care delivery.

Relational interventions

These involve the use of education-based activities in the form of interprofessional learning interventions or practice-based activities in the form of team checklists and interprofessional team meetings. All of these approaches are examples of direct teamwork interventions.

Interprofessional learning activities

Working effectively as a member of a health or social care team is a complicated task (see Chapter 4). Despite this complexity, most practitioners continue to receive little or no formal training or education to work within an interprofessional team. A growing number of interprofessional learning activities have, however, been developed and implemented across care settings. We describe below three interprofessional learning activities: team training, simulation and team retreats.

Team training interventions: These consist of interactive workshops or educational sessions in which students and/or practitioners come together in teams to discuss their collaborative work and problem-solve. Such interventions usually involve a combination of practice-based and classroom-based experiences, focusing on preparing students for future teamwork interactions (see Box 6.1) or enhancing team members' existing teamwork abilities (e.g. Reeves *et al.*, 2006).

Box 6.1   Interprofessional team training intervention.

Nisbet *et al.* (2008) describe a study of an interprofessional team intervention implemented across the medical, nursing and allied health professional programmes in Australia. The intervention was ten hours in total, delivered over 4 weeks and included the participation of 16 senior-level students from medicine, nursing, nutrition and dietetics, occupational therapy, physiotherapy, social work and speech pathology. The activities in which students participated included team building exercises, observations of another profession's procedures, patient case discussions, ward meetings as well as periods of reflection on team performance. The authors report that the students showed a greater understanding of interprofessional teamwork and positive attitudes towards working in an interprofessional team following the intervention.

On occasion, such training can be delivered to students and practitioners jointly to encourage discussion and reflection among individuals at different stages in their development (e.g. Taylor *et al.*, 2001; Boyce *et al.*, 2009). Increasingly, such interventions involve patients and their families who interact with professionals and/or students to provide a patient perspective on the delivery of care (e.g. Weingart *et al.*, 2009).

Simulation: A recent development in teamwork interventions is the use of simulated learning experiences. These range from low-fidelity (role-play exercises) to high-fidelity (computerised manikins, simulated clinical environments) activities. Simulated learning opportunities are regarded as advantageous as they allow students and qualified professionals to practice teamwork in ways that approximate actual clinical work as well as time to reflect upon their shared experiences. Typically, high-fidelity team simulation learning activities are offered in emergency, intensive care or operating room settings (e.g. Anderson and Leflore, 2008). There is growing evidence for the effects of such team-based simulated learning. For example, Wisborg *et al.* (2008) evaluated the impact of a trauma team training initiative designed to improve knowledge and skills in resuscitation. The study found that increases in knowledge and confidence were reported by team members from 26 hospitals, and these increases were maintained after 6 months. Other examples of simulated learning include the interprofessional management of emergencies, in which simulated disasters have been developed to help improve interprofessional team performance and increase the efficiency of care systems in an emergency or pandemic situation (Centennial College, 2009; Jeffs *et al.*, in review).

Team retreats: At times teams are invited to retreats in which they reflect on and/or plan their collaborative work away from the distractions of clinical practice. While it is argued that such interventions help to ensure that members are 'distanced' from the pressures of everyday life, they may also generate a problem of dislocation. As members are apart from the real world, any learning that occurs at retreats may be left behind when they return to practice. Long (1996) provides a useful example in her study of a 2-day residential team building workshop held for primary health care teams in the UK. This intervention aimed to improve the understanding of different professional roles and how members could enhance their collaborative work. Interviews conducted before and after the workshops indicated that most participants felt there was more agreement over team goals. However, it was also felt that interprofessional friction between certain team members was unaltered, when they returned to clinical practice.

While evidence from systematic reviews has indicated that interprofessional learning can result in short-term gains regarding collaborative knowledge, skills and attitudes (e.g. Hammick *et al.*, 2007), the long-term sustainability of these gains needs further exploration.

Communication interventions

In general, these direct teamwork interventions employ two main (practice-based) approaches: the use of meetings or rounds and the use of checklists or briefing sheets to help enhance interprofessional communication.

Team checklists: These can help team members focus on the often routine tasks they need to perform together. Checklists can also help trigger communication and dialogue between members, which can in turn improve their relationships. Box 6.2 provides an example of a communication intervention for surgical teams which uses a simple checklist to improve safety and relations.

The use of checklists has grown in recent years, mainly due to the emphasis on patient safety (see Chapter 2). Checklists can vary in nature, from simple tools such as that outlined in Box 6.2 to more comprehensive tools such as the SBAR (Situation–Background–Assessment–Recommendation), which aims to provide team members with a framework for communication around a patient's condition (Leonard *et al.*, 2004).

Box 6.2 A team communication intervention.

Lingard *et al.* (2005) developed and also studied the implementation of a preoperative checklist to support a team briefing in the operating room (OR) and assessed whether the briefing reduced communication failures. During each briefing the OR team members were gathered together by the research facilitator to review the upcoming surgical case. The checklist contained prompts for patient-related information (e.g. allergies) and procedural-related information (e.g. equipment, patient positioning and anaesthetic needs). The team members shared their knowledge and resolved any knowledge gaps or assumptions about the case in a brief 'huddle' triggered by the items of the checklist. Local clinical champions were key to the implementation of the checklist. The timing of the briefing was important and the coordination of the team members was the biggest challenge. Workflow also presented a major barrier in bringing the team together since the three professions in the OR team could follow distinct workflow patterns that might take them in various directions in the pre-operative period.

Team meetings: The other main communication intervention is team meetings, which attempt to improve awareness and understanding of team member's roles, responsibilities and shared goals. Curley *et al.* (1998) provided a useful example of this type of intervention in their study of the introduction of weekly interprofessional rounds to promote communication among physicians, nurses, a pharmacist, a nutritionist and a social worker in an acute care setting in the US. More recently, Aston *et al.* (2005) described the development and implementation of a surgical morning meeting designed to improve communication between physicians and nurses based in a paediatric hospital in Australia. The researchers gathered qualitative data in the form of semi-structured interviews and found that these meetings were highly valued. It was also found that the meetings helped plan the day's activities and contributed to better interprofessional relations.

Processual interventions

These interventions aim to improve teamwork by organising the nature of work undertaken by interprofessional teams. They span four broad (practice-based) approaches: crew resource management (CRM), integrated care pathways, case management and role shifting. While CRM is an example of a direct teamwork intervention, integrated care pathways, case management and role shifting are all examples of indirect teamwork interventions.

Crew resource management

CRM is an approach which emerged from the airline industry and that aimed to improve safety among airline crews by providing explicit, detailed written procedures which cover a range of potential situations and problems that crews may face in the cockpit (Salas et al., 2001) (see Chapter 3). The approach helps ensure that tasks and their allocation to different members of the crew are clear. It is usually offered collectively to flight crews to ensure that each member knows their own tasks and those of their colleagues, as well as to ensure that work is carried out in a collaborative fashion. As we noted earlier, this approach has been employed by a number of health and social care organisations to help reduce error by interprofessional teams, usually in acute care settings.

Studies on the use of CRM interventions in health and social care have indicated that it can achieve some gains such as improvements in team function (Risser et al., 1999) and some reductions in the frequency and severity of adverse events (Morey et al., 2002; Pratt et al., 2007). However, as we noted previously the gains are generally modest and the use of CRM to promote teamwork in health and social care settings can encounter challenges, especially where tasks are unpredictable or where the team works across a number of locations.

Integrated care pathways

Integrated care pathways – also called critical paths, collaborative care plans and multidisciplinary action plans – are interventions in which the events and activities involved in a patient's care trajectory are specified within a certain time period. The aim is to standardise the delivery of care, the length of stay and the clinical management of the patient. Ignatavicius and Hausman (1995) refer to integrated care pathways as interprofessional plans of care that outline the optimal sequencing and timing of interventions for patients with a particular diagnosis, procedure or symptom. As such, the pathways depend upon ongoing communication, teamwork and the commitment to deliver integrated care between professionals. Box 6.3 describes a study which evaluated the use of an integrated care pathway on interprofessional teamwork within an orthopaedic setting.

Box 6.3   An integrated care pathway intervention.

Atwal and Caldwell (2002) employed an action research design in which they worked with practitioners to implement and evaluate an integrated care pathway for patients with fractured neck of femurs in a UK teaching hospital. The study explored whether such pathways enhanced and developed interprofessional teamwork and collaboration and enabled effective flow of information between the professionals and across the organisation. Data were gathered in the form of stakeholder interviews, interprofessional audit and analysis of divergence from the integrated care pathway. Findings revealed that the introduction of the pathway did result in some improvements in clinical processes and outcomes. The pathway enabled professionals to identify why discharge delays had occurred and also helped to coordinate care. However, the pathway did not result in an overall improvement in team processes or interprofessional relations. The authors concluded that while the introduction of an integrated care protocol can help improve the delivery of care, this intervention alone did not equip professionals with the skills to become competent interprofessional team players.

While it has been argued that integrated care pathways provide a potentially valuable approach to delivering interprofessional care in teams (e.g. Leathard, 2003b), they are limited to relatively simple and predictable patient conditions. As a result, they can only be employed for a small fraction of the work undertaken by interprofessional teams.

Case management

Case management is an intervention which involves a single professional (typically a nurse or a social worker), or sometimes a lay person with specific training, who takes responsibility for, and coordinates patient care by liaison and collaboration with other health and social care professionals. Case management helps to ensure that patients are admitted and transitioned to the appropriate level of care, have an effective plan of care and receive appropriate treatment by the team of professionals involved in their care. It has been a popular intervention in the delivery of mental health care (e.g. Ziguras and Stuart, 2000) and the management of chronic illnesses such as diabetes (e.g. Norris *et al.*, 2002) and is a good example of an indirect teamwork intervention. (Its primary aim is to promote the delivery of well-coordinated care, through the use of a single individual who works to coordinate the activities of their colleagues).

Role shifting

Role shifting encompasses three main interventions: role substitution, role delegation and role creation (see Chapter 4). Role substitution involves one profession assuming the tasks normally undertaken by another. In the case of the introduction of the nurse practitioner role, this can be seen as an expansion of nursing into the realm traditionally occupied by medicine. Role delegation usually involves a profession handing over typically 'low-status' tasks they have traditionally undertaken. Examples include nurses delegating work to health care assistants (Spilsbury and Meyer, 2004) and occupational therapists delegating to occupational therapy assistants (Nancarrow and Mackey, 2005).

New role interventions – in the form of the introduction of a new professional or non-professional role – can be used to support existing interprofessional teamwork and collaboration activities. For instance, a care coordinator role (a role undertaken by non-professional health care worker) was introduced into an acute care directorate to coordinate the work of a number of professions such as physicians, nurses and social workers (Bridges *et al.*, 2003). While care coordinators were found to be successful in helping the professions communicate and in providing more coordinated care, their role was also perceived to overlap with nursing and social work areas, especially when working to coordinate the discharge of patients.

As Box 6.4 indicates, the introduction of a new role, community pharmacists, into primary care teams resulted in some interprofessional tensions.

Box 6.4   Introducing a new role into primary care.

Dobson *et al.* (2006) surveyed the introduction of community pharmacists into interprofessional primary care teams in Canada. Traditionally, community pharmacists have practised in privately owned businesses. However, recent health and social care reforms encouraged greater involvement of community-based pharmacists within primary care teams. Nearly 500 questionnaires were returned. Most respondents agreed that community pharmacists should be part of the interprofessional primary care team. Overall, community pharmacists responded that they had a positive working relationship with physicians, who were willing to work with them to share patient information and to seek their advice. However, the pharmacists also indicated that a number of factors that impeded their work, such as time to carry out team activities, opportunities to meet and get to know members of other professions, the adequacy of financial reimbursement as well as a tendency of other professions to protect their professional boundaries.

Organisational interventions

These interventions focus on improving teamwork at the organisational level. We found three types that have been employed (indirectly) to enhance teamwork – quality improvement teams, accreditation and reorganising the delivery of care.

Quality improvement

Quality improvement assumes that individuals work and learn together to collectively improve the quality of their work environment and the products or services they provide (see Chapter 3). Continuous quality improvement (CQI) and total quality management (TQM) initiatives are commonly employed within health and social care organisations. These involve teams coming together to review a 'problem' they have identified and often employ a PDSA (plan, do, study and act) cycle to improve their approach to care delivery (e.g. Gazarian *et al.*, 2001). Studies have indicated that the use of CQI approaches can help improve staff morale and enhance collaboration and the quality of the care (e.g. Treadwell *et al.*, 2002; Wilcock *et al.*, 2002).

However, as we discussed in Chapter 3, the applicability of QI approaches to health and social care settings has its limits. While studies have indicated that the use of such interventions can improve the quality of service delivery through the use of teams, often little attention is paid to attempting to improve the quality of team performances or interprofessional processes.

Accreditation

Accreditation is a QI approach in which a certification of certain standards is awarded by an accrediting body. Accreditation sets standards and monitors the quality of teamwork which occurs within a team or an institution. An example is provided by the Magnet Hospital initiative (see Box 1.6), which has been accredited by the American Nurses Association's Creditentialing Center. Studies have reported some gains in relation to lower mortality rates (Aiken *et al.*, 1994) and better interprofessional relations (Aiken *et al.*, 2008), when compared with non-Magnet hospitals. However, it is unclear whether the crediting process has resulted in a wide range of organisations adopting this approach.

Other examples of accreditation include the Quality Assurance Agency in the UK (see Chapter 2) and the Accreditation of Interprofessional Health Education in Canada (Association of Facilities of Medicine of Canada, 2007), which aim to provide accreditation for higher education institutions involved in the delivery of interprofessional education experiences.

Reorganising the delivery of care

A further way to intervene to improve the quality of interprofessional teamwork is by changing the way care is organised within a specific department or clinic. Such interventions usually involve health service managers working with professionals to introduce new organisational policies or procedures which aim to, for instance, integrate the way care is delivered by different groups of professionals. We give an example later (see Chapter 8) of an organisational intervention which aimed to enhance interprofessional teamwork and collaboration. This intervention attempted to reorganise the delivery of medical care through a new patient triage system which ensured that physicians' patients were allocated to specific wards to facilitate better collaboration with nurses, therapists, pharmacists and social workers.

Contextual interventions

Contextual-level interventions are broader in scope. Their implementation depends upon governments and/or professional regulatory bodies, intervening in the form of policies that directly foster teamwork or through funding to support the development of local interprofessional activities.

Policy initiatives

Government and professional regulatory body policies have played an important role in the promotion of interprofessional teamwork in a number of countries (e.g. Department of Health, 1997; Association of American Medical Colleges, 2009) (see Chapter 2). The effects of these national and international policies can be profound. For example, calls for increased patient safety have resulted in the establishment of a number of publicly funded patient safety agencies around the world (e.g. the National Patient Safety Agency in the UK and the Australian Patient Safety Foundation) which all advocate for the use of teamwork to improve the delivery of safe, error-free care. Similarly, calls for improvements in the education and training of professionals to develop teamwork attributes have resulted in a worldwide response by educators to deliver a wide range of pre- and post-qualifying interprofessional education activities (e.g. Barr *et al.*, 2005).

Funding interventions

Funding interventions to promote the development, implementation and evaluation of interprofessional teamwork are the second type of contextual intervention. In the US, for example, funding by the W.K. Kellogg Foundation was key to developing and implementing a range of interprofessional team initiatives (see Chapter 1). Boxes 2.2 and 2.3 provide additional examples of interventions which aimed to provide funding for the development and evaluation of interprofessional teamwork in the UK and Canada.

Multifaceted interventions

Interventions, such as team training, applied alone may be ineffective in achieving changes in teamwork. They may, however, usefully form part of a multifaceted intervention in which individual activities are strengthened and reinforced, for example, by an organisational intervention aimed to support teamwork practice or the introduction of a new checklist to support team communication. There are a number of examples of such multifaceted interventions. For instance, Morey *et al.* (2002) describe an emergency department teamwork intervention which included team training to reduce errors and improve performance, coaching and mentoring of teamwork behaviours, introduction of whiteboards to enhance information exchange and reconfiguration of workspace to help team members interact more easily. Box 6.5 provides another example of a multifaceted intervention.

Box 6.5 A multifaceted teamwork intervention based in general medicine.

Vogwill (2008) describes a study that employed a multifaceted intervention to improve the quality of communication exchange during interprofessional working within a general medicine context. The intervention consisted of three strands of activity: eliciting management support, the use of team-based consensus building and problem-solving, and the introduction of a nurse charged with the responsibility for leading interprofessional rounds and co-ordinating care. An evaluation was undertaken to understand the content and communication processes of interprofessional meetings, and the needs of the participants. The results indicated that information loss decreased after the intervention. Nevertheless, physicians reported they were not satisfied with information exchange with nurses. In addition, while the nurses felt that interprofessional rounds helped to support communication between nurses and physicians, these views were not shared by staff physicians. Overall, the results suggest that even after use of this multifaceted intervention, there were still many interprofessional communication problems.

Other multifaceted interventions include those described by Friedman and Berger (2004). This team intervention consisted of education to improve definitions of team member roles; the use of daily meetings between physicians, case managers and charge nurses; and the introduction of a monthly meeting for the entire team to discuss their interprofessional work. Horak *et al.* (2004) also introduced a range of educational, relational and organisational interventions to improve teamwork between physicians, nurses, social workers, dietitians and physical therapists.

Summarising teamwork interventions

Table 6.1 provides a summary of teamwork interventions and their reported effects on interprofessional teamwork, based on the limited evaluation work available.

While we have not undertaken a systematic review of the effects of these interventions, Table 6.1 indicates, based on the studies we included, that in general the reported effects of many of these interventions are limited. Also, this table indicates that most teamwork interventions are indirect in nature – improvements in teamwork are usually a secondary goal within a wider programme of enhancing the delivery of care.

Table 6.1 Summarising interprofessional team interventions.

Intervention	Focus	Type	Description	Effects on teamwork
Interprofessional learning activities	Relational	Direct	Team training, simulation, team retreats	Short-term changes to individual attitudes, knowledge and skills
Communication interventions	Relational	Direct	Team checklists, team meetings/rounds	Some improvement in interprofessional communication
Crew resource management	Processual	Direct	Focus on clarity of tasks and task allocation	Can contribute to improved team function and some reduction in errors
Integrated care pathways	Processual	Indirect	Standardisation of care process	Some improvements in team function and patient outcomes
Case management	Processual	Indirect	Single professional coordinating work of others	Some use in coordinating clinical work; little effect on quality of teamwork
Role shifting	Processual	Indirect	Substitution, delegation, introduction of new roles	Variable – often professional overlap can occur
Quality improvement	Organisational	Indirect, though can be direct	CQI, TQM, PDSA cycle	Some improvement in team process and quality of care
Accreditation	Organisational	Indirect	Accrediting organisations and learning activities	Some improvement in collaboration between medicine and nursing
Reorganising care	Organisational	Direct and indirect	Introduction of policies and procedures, changing working patterns	Can help improve team communication
Policy changes	Context	Direct and/or indirect	Policies that create teamwork incentives	Increases attention and intervention activity
Funding	Context	Direct and/or indirect	Changing financial arrangements and funds for teamwork	Increases attention and intervention activity
Multifaceted	Any two or more of the above	Direct and/or indirect	Can employ team training, checklists, CQI, etc.	Can contribute to improvements in team organisation and team relations

Current limitations

The teamwork interventions that we have presented share a number of similar limitations, as discussed below.

Poor intervention design

Few of the interventions we reviewed were based on an empirical, research-based understanding of the problem they were attempting to address. As a consequence of an intuitive rather than an empirical approach, many interventions tackled problems in a naïve way. For instance, relational interventions, such as team checklists and interprofessional meetings, ignored 'higher order' (structural) problems such as imbalances in interprofessional relations and inequalities in power. As Long (1996) found in her evaluation of an interprofessional retreat for primary health team members, despite reporting some gains with regard to team functioning, 'traditional hierarchical relations' (p. 940) created by financial and status inequalities between the physicians and other team members were largely untouched. Indeed, for Funnell (1995), such interventions usually overlook the contradiction which exists between their need for a shared approach and the way professions operate – in a largely autonomous fashion. As Funnell argued:

> By directing attention towards the need for an educational solution to greater service co-ordination, it also diverts discussion from the appropriateness or not of existing professional [. . .] boundaries. (p. 165)

In addition, we found that few interventions were explicitly based upon theory. Grol et al. (2007) argue in their review of theories for use in health care interventions that making explicit the theoretical assumptions behind the choice of interventions is important for a number of reasons. For example, theory can offer a generalisable framework for considering effectiveness across different clinical contexts. Also, basing interventions on theoretical assumptions helps prevent important social, organisational and professional factors from being overlooked.

Intervening with 'magical thinking'

The past few years have seen the growing employment by health and social care institutions of consultants to 'intervene' in the workplace order to provide 'solutions' to poor interprofessional team relations. Box 6.6 is the announcement for a recent talk given by a consultant to a health and social care audience.

> **Box 6.6**   An example of a consultant-led intervention.
>
> A specialist in constraints management will speak about 'The Evaporating Cloud' – one of the six thinking processes in the theory of constraints to enable the focused improvement of systems. The 'Evaporating Cloud' is suited to finding a solution to virtually any problem. It creates breakthrough solutions by going a step beyond root cause analysis. This results in win-win solutions that avoid compromises and break through seemingly impossible situations.

An increasingly popular approach used by consultants attempting to offer solutions to teamwork problems is 'appreciative inquiry', which encourages individuals to adopt a positive approach to managing change. However, this type of inquiry has been criticised for its lack of critical analysis and oversight of pre-existing structural social, economic and political imbalances (e.g. Grant and Humphries, 2006). As Salaman (2002) has argued, the language of personal empowerment used within appreciative inquiry creates the appearance of democratic change while removing from view any critical analysis of the current status quo in relation to existing social and economic inequalities.

For us, the use of such approaches to intervene in teams is problematic. They not only overlook the complexity inherent in interprofessional teams, but also divert attention from the inequalities which can bedevil teamwork. As such, they provide examples of 'magical thinking' – whereby real world thinking is replaced with notions of *make-believe* (Malinowski, 1948).

Conclusions and implications

Different interventions – relational, processual, organisational and contextual – have been employed to improve interprofessional teamwork directly or indirectly. Most are single interventions while a few employ a multifaceted approach. Encouragingly, this latter type of intervention appears to hold some promise for affecting interprofessional teamwork in a number of ways. However, we found that the development of most teamwork interventions was based on little, if any, prior empirical work. As a result, most interventions overlooked structural factors which can impede efforts to improve teamwork. While the use, development and implementation of interventions to improve teamwork have made some useful progress, there is still some way to go. In particular, interventions require further thought on their form, content and delivery. They also need to be evaluated rigorously to better understand their effects on team relations, processes of care and patient outcomes.

theory, account for individual and team-level performance, capture team processes and outcomes, and adhere to standards for methodological quality.

Why evaluate?

Given the concerns outlined above, careful and thoughtful evaluation of interprofessional teamwork activities and initiatives is essential.

For example, evaluation can help to:

- Understand the nature of teamwork, including how and why it works or has no effects
- Identify those situations where one form of teamwork is more (or less) effective than others
- Provide accountability for health and social care resources to those who provide or control them – regional/national authorities, research and service funders, consumers and foundations
- Strengthen the organisations in which evaluations are conducted, through building capacity for improvement and enhancing effectiveness and efficiency
- Provide generalisable evidence which can assist in advancing knowledge in the field.

Without the insights and evidence from evaluations, resources may be wasted on ineffective, or even harmful teamwork interventions. As a result, funders and commissioning bodies may in the longer term become less supportive of efforts to promote teamwork. Our goal is therefore to encourage practitioners, managers and researchers to build an informative and reliable evidence base for improving care and patient outcomes through interprofessional teamwork.

What is evaluation?

Evaluation has been defined as a process of 'appraising human activities in a formal, systematic way' (Kelly, 2004, p. 523). Similarly, Patton saw evaluation as 'any effort to *increase human effectiveness* through systematic data-based enquiry' (Patton, 1990, p. 11). A key purpose of evaluation is to make judgements about the usefulness of health and social programmes. Evaluation is therefore focused on assessing change in activities or programmes; addresses pre-specified questions in a transparent way; and is based on the systematic collection and analysis of data.

Evaluation is an empirical activity in which inquiry is made into the causes and effects of actions. Evaluations, as we discuss, may be quantitative or qualitative or utilise both approaches. A number of qualitative and quantitative components may be assembled to provide a complete picture of the effects of a teamwork intervention. Comparisons between different actions (or interventions) aimed at the same goal (or outcome) can show comparative effectiveness in achieving that goal or outcome. For example, in a randomised control trial undertaken by Wild *et al.* (2004), patients of a ward in a community hospital were randomised to either the intervention medical team, which conducted daily interprofessional rounds, or to the control team, which provided standard care. The effects of these two different actions on length of hospital stay were measured. The study found no difference in length of hospital stay between the intervention and control groups.

Evaluators may also explore the experiences of those who undertake, or are the recipients of, teamwork in order to reveal the meanings and values attributed to it. For example, a qualitative study was undertaken to evaluate the first specialist adolescent cancer unit established in the UK (Mulhall *et al.*, 2004). The evaluation aimed to explore the culture of the unit; the experiences of patients and their parents as well as the views of staff delivering care in the unit, who constituted a cancer team. Both semi-structured interviews with these groups and observations of routine unit activities were undertaken. Mulhall and colleagues reported a range of findings, including that the availability of an expert group of health care providers was key to ensuring an appropriate care environment. The authors concluded that the complex health care needs of adolescents with cancer may best be met by teams working in specialist units.

In addition, evaluators may examine the costs of teamwork actions or programmes so as to inform decisions regarding their cost-effectiveness. For example, an economic analysis was undertaken alongside a trial of assertive community treatment for homeless adults with severe mental illnesses in the US (Lehman *et al.*, 1999). The effects of this treatment, which promoted continuity of care and was delivered by an interprofessional team, were compared with usual care. The main outcome was the number of days of stable community housing enjoyed by participants. Lehman and colleagues concluded that the assertive community treatment intervention was more effective but not more costly than usual care for increasing time spent in stable housing by adults with severe mental illnesses.

Interventions to improve the process of interprofessional teamworking and to maximise its benefits are complex and are often composed of many different elements. Consequently, evaluations of these interventions are frequently multi-faceted. To help understand this complexity, we categorise evaluations according to their *purpose*, the *targets* of action and the *types of evidence* that evaluators may gather.

Evaluation purpose

The purpose of an evaluation may be to provide formative information, summative information or both. An evaluation that is undertaken early in the development of a new or modified teamwork intervention may be useful in understanding the context in which an intervention is to be implemented as well as in improving its design. At this stage of development, there is a need to incorporate feedback from a range of stakeholders in order to improve the ongoing design and delivery of the intervention. Evaluation for this purpose is *formative* in that it contributes to shaping an intervention or its implementation.

Once the final form of the intervention is defined and implemented, the focus of evaluation may shift towards such issues as the overall worth of the new approach, including its effectiveness and efficiency, in comparison with usual care, existing approaches or alternatives. Such evaluations may be conducted at the site where the intervention was implemented initially, or more widely, at other sites. Evaluation for this purpose is *summative* and may include data on:

- Perceptions of those participating in and experiencing care within the new model of teamwork – often using qualitative approaches
- Processes of care that have changed as a consequence of the intervention – often using both qualitative and quantitative approaches
- Impacts on practitioners, resource use or patient outcomes – often quantitative and may include economic data.

Box 7.1 provides two examples of evaluation studies – one which employed a formative approach and the other which employed a summative approach.

Box 7.1   Examples of formative and summative evaluations.

Formative evaluation. Onyskiw *et al.* (1999) describe an interprofessional community-based child abuse prevention project which was the focus of a formative evaluation of a project implementation. The evaluation used a qualitative approach including semi structured interviews and client record review. The findings suggested that clients particularly valued the informal support received from team members. In addition, clients found the community-based approach of the initiative and the collaborative nature of the project team beneficial. Clients also appreciated the availability of support when it was needed and the quick responses of the team. The authors concluded that interprofessional community-based models of service delivery can contribute to a more effective response to families in need. They noted that the factors identified as important in this formative evaluation could help others to develop similar programmes or improve their current programmes.

Summative evaluation. A large RCT, involving 33 nursing homes (15 assigned to the experimental group and 18 to the control group), was conducted by Schmidt *et al.* (1998) to examine the effects of monthly facilitated team rounds on the quality and quantity of psychotropic drug prescribing. Participants in the team rounds included physicians, pharmacists, nurses and nursing assistants. Rounds were led by a pharmacist and took place once a month over a period of 12 months. The trial found that the average number of drugs prescribed in the experimental homes was the same before and after the intervention whereas the average number of drugs increased significantly in the control homes. The authors concluded that monthly team meetings improved prescribing of psychotropic drugs in nursing homes.

Target of the evaluation

Evaluations can also be grouped on the basis of their target or targets. An evaluation of an interprofessional teamwork intervention may be focused on the inputs to the programme; the processes through which the intervention is implemented; the intervention outcomes; or the wider impacts of the programme. Examples of evaluation areas related to different targets are shown in Table 7.1.

Table 7.1   Teamwork evaluation questions for different teamwork activities.

Intervention target	Areas to evaluate
Inputs	These may be the training experiences, consultations and new staff added to a team in order to achieve desired improvements in teamwork
Processes	Changes in work process, especially with regard to interactions among the team members
Outcomes	These relate to the goals of the teamwork intervention and the extent to which the intervention has: - Changed, increased or improved collaboration - Made communication more informative and less interruptive - Resulted in more appropriate and inclusive consultation and decision-making
Impacts	These relate to the goals of care delivered by an interprofessional team: - How and to what extent have changes been achieved in aspects of their lives that patients value (e.g. health status, social integration, probability of remaining in home environment, length of stay)? - To what extent have staff and teamwork life improved, as measured by changes such as job satisfaction, work stress or staff turnover?

Types of evidence needed

When considering how to evaluate a teamwork intervention, a key question is whether *local evidence* or *generalisable evidence* is required. To understand the usual effects of teamwork interventions in particular setting, and to understand the factors that modify those effects, generalisable evidence is required (Lewin *et al.*, 2009b). Such evidence may also help to generate and test theories that offer insights into fundamental elements of teamworking. High quality intervention studies, such as RCTs, are a robust way of generating such evidence. We discuss this type of evaluation in more detail below.

Local evidence or knowledge 'that is available from the specific setting or settings in which a policy decision and action will be taken' (Lewin *et al.*, 2009b) is often used, alongside other forms of evidence, to improve local care and inform local health policy decisions. Local evidence is only useful to clinicians, managers and policy makers responsible for delivering and improving care in a local institution or setting. While generalisable evidence is needed to draw overall conclusions about the effects of teamwork interventions, local evidence is needed for most decisions about what actions should be taken. Local evidence may be obtained from routine information systems in hospitals or health authorities or from research that has collected or analysed data on a local level. The range of local evidence needed will depend on the nature of the teamwork issue being addressed. Box 7.2 outlines some of the ways that local knowledge may be used to inform decisions regarding teamworking.

Box 7.2   Uses of local knowledge in understanding or improving teamworking (adapted from Lewin *et al.*, 2009b).

Local knowledge can be used to:

- Diagnose the likely causes of a problem that may be related to inadequate interprofessional teamworking
- Estimate the size of a problem that may be a consequence of inadequate teamworking or communication between professionals
- Contextualise evidence from global reviews of the effects of interventions to improve collaboration between professionals
- Describe care delivery, financial or governance arrangements in a setting in which a teamwork intervention is being considered
- Inform assessments of the likely impacts of different options for addressing a problem related to inadequate interprofessional teamworking
- Inform judgements about values and preferences regarding teamwork options (i.e. the relative importance that individuals attach to possible impacts of these options) and views regarding these options
- Estimate the costs (and savings) of teamwork interventions
- Assess the availability of resources (including human resources, technical capacity, infrastructure, equipment) needed to implement an intervention to improve teamworking
- Identify barriers to implementing interventions to improving communication between professionals
- Monitor the sustainability of a teamwork programme over time

---

Much evidence is both local and generalisable. For example, a high quality evaluation may address a local question regarding the effects of an intervention as well as contribute to generalisable, global knowledge on effectiveness. It has been argued that such global knowledge is the best starting point for judgements about the effects of programmes and factors that modify those effects, and for insights into ways to explore and address problems (Oxman *et al.*, 2009). This type of evidence can be applied across a range of settings by clinicians and managers working in settings outside those in which the original study was conducted. Such evidence is, of course, also of interest to researchers who aim to develop theories about how teams work, and their effects on care as well as in compiling global evidence on the effects of an intervention (such as within a systematic review, see for example, Stroke Unit Trialists, 2007; Zwarenstein *et al.*, 2009).

All evaluations of teamwork interventions should aim to use the most rigorous evaluation methods feasible within resource constraints. Those taking decisions about the implementation of teamwork initiatives should be cautious about using only local evidence to assess their possible impact. Local evidence may seem to be more directly relevant than studies conducted in other settings and is likely to describe what has occurred in that setting in an understandable and usable way. However, such evidence may be less reliable (Lewin *et al.*, 2009b).

Types of evaluation

In this section we discuss three types of evaluation which can be employed to study the nature and/or effects of interprofessional teamwork interventions: quantitative, qualitative and mixed methods evaluations.

Quantitative evaluation

There are two main types of quantitative evaluation: descriptive and intervention studies. Descriptive studies (also sometimes called observational studies) use numbers to describe the variations in a phenomenon across different instances. Intervention studies are experiments in which an intervention (such as team training) is allocated randomly to some but not other groups and the effects on specific outcomes then monitored.

Descriptive studies

Quantitative descriptive studies do not actively intervene in care delivery, nor do they implement any changes to the way in which teams operate. Instead, they aim to measure the impact of different approaches or interventions by looking at and comparing existing processes and outcomes in different units or settings. In this sense, these are observations of 'natural' experiments. Descriptive studies rely on the allocation of interventions which may have occurred differently in different settings. This may be by design (of someone other than the evaluator), by chance or by some other factor, such as regional incentives, regulations or cultural tendencies.

In these studies, the investigator does not allocate the different interventions or approaches in a fashion designed to minimise variation between the groups receiving these interventions. There may therefore be profound differences between the sites, settings or people receiving the contrasting interventions. These differences might well explain any variation in outcomes measured. The risk in descriptive research is that conclusions on the usefulness of contrasting approaches to the organisation and support of teamwork may be based upon confusion between cause and result. Confounding differences between the sites or people receiving the intervention may prevent valid conclusions on effectiveness from being drawn. The threat to validity is sufficiently great that we recommend against this type of evaluation as a way of drawing conclusions on the *effectiveness* of teamwork interventions. At best, descriptive studies may generate a *hypothesis* that a particular form of teamwork or intervention to promote teamwork might result in improved outcomes. Further studies would then be needed to generate evidence to confirm or deny this hypothesis.

Intervention studies

Many interventions are ineffective and/or may lead to a waste of resources. Information whether interventions are effective or not can inform future design and delivery. Two categories of intervention study – randomised and non-randomised – can be employed. Both are discussed below.

Non-randomised designs: These studies do not employ randomisation in the allocation of an intervention, such as team training, to individuals (such as nurses or physicians) or groups (such as ward teams). Before-and-after studies, controlled before-and-after studies and interrupted time series studies are all examples of non-randomised designs (see Appendix 2). In general, they require fewer resources and are more easily conducted on a small scale or in a single institution. However, the validity of the results that they produce is substantially lower than in randomised studies. This is partly because they are often more subject to bias than randomised trials and, partly because they are designed and analysed with less attention to statistical science.

Randomised designs: These studies randomise units (such as individuals or teams) to either receive an intervention or not; receiving instead either 'usual care' or an alternative activity). RCTs are considered the gold standard for assessing causality, and for evaluating the impact of an intervention (Grimshaw *et al.*, 2004). This is because they are effective at reducing many potential causes of bias, and thus of invalid evaluation results. Randomisation is crucial as it reduces:

- Allocation bias (by removing control of allocation of the intervention from the investigator)
- Measurement bias (by standardising measurement in intervention and control groups)
- Chance (through careful and appropriate sample size calculation)
- Confounding (the probability that some known or unknown influence may affect outcomes).

Establishing validity

The type of evidence needed (e.g. local or generalisable), and the resources available, drive most choices in evaluation design. The first goal of a quantitative evaluation though is to ensure internal validity – the degree to which an observed effect can be attributed to the intervention under study. Its second goal is to maximise external validity or generalisability. Generalisability, also known as applicability refers to the degree to which the results of a study in one setting can be applied to others. If a study has poor internal validity, that is the relationship between intervention and impact has not been accurately measured, it cannot have external validity. This is because the question of whether this spurious finding represents what would happen in other settings is moot. By contrast, a study of an intervention in one setting may produce valid results for that setting, though its results may not be widely applicable. We first discuss the elements of study design which establish internal validity and then those elements which establish external validity.

There are many reasons why an intervention may appear effective, when it is not. For example, a treatment for the common cold may seem to work because a person is cured a few days after taking it. The clinical improvement may be due to the effect of the treatment or the natural course of a self-limiting disease that lasts only a few days. Similarly, teamwork in a given department may improve after an interprofessional intervention, but it could improve for several reasons, including that the teamwork was already improving or additional funding resulted in the recruitment of extra staff around the time of the intervention.

The types of studies mentioned above vary in their ability to control for bias and ascertain whether an observed effect is the result of the intervention in question. However, even a perfectly valid study may not allow us to determine the degree to which a result is relevant to *real world* conditions. That is, if a result found in one setting could be reproduced in regular practice, outside an RCT (Grimshaw and Eccles, 2004). Pragmatic RCTs (i.e. those designed to find out about the effectiveness of interventions in routine, everyday practice) are designed to maximise the relevance of the results for real world decision-making, and often for a broad range of settings (Thorpe *et al.*, 2009). Expanding a successful pilot programme to the regional or national level may not produce similar results unless efforts are taken to maximise the generalisability or external validity of the study. Pragmatic RCTs are the appropriate design for such expansions from pilot to large-scale real world testing.

Limitations

There are, of course, a number of limitations associated with undertaking quantitative evaluation. Experimental studies such as RCTs, which compare groups with and without the intervention, can tell us about the effects of an intervention. However, they cannot provide answers to *why* these effects occurred. In addition, a common criticism of quantitative approaches is that they are highly reductive. For example, the use of such designs may be seen as reducing complicated social phenomena, such as interprofessional teamwork, into a range of simplistic variables to facilitate measurement. As we discuss below, use of mixed methods evaluations that employ both quantitative and qualitative approaches can overcome some of these limitations.

Qualitative evaluation

The use of qualitative methods is grounded in the social sciences. Qualitative approaches attempt to describe and interpret human phenomena rather than measure them (Green and Thorogood, 2004). These methods focus on finding answers to questions centred on social experience, including the values and perceptions of individuals and groups, and how they experience the world around them, including health care. Qualitative methods have particular strengths within evaluation including understanding how and why effects come about; exploring participants' experiences of phenomena; explaining intervention outcomes in relation to social and organisational contexts; and examining how interventions might be improved.

Qualitative methods tend to be used more for formative than for summative evaluation. They usually focus on:

- Developing and piloting of interventions
- Understanding intervention processes (e.g. how they are implemented and received by participants)
- Investigating the outcome and impact of interventions
- Theory building.

We discuss each of these in more detail below.

Developing and piloting interventions

Qualitative approaches to evaluation may be used to develop and pilot new health and social care initiatives by exploring their processes and effects. This is particularly useful for complex health and social care issues (e.g. Oakley *et al.*, 2006), such as those directed at changing the behaviours of professionals who work in interprofessional teams. These studies are often small scale, and may focus on an exploration of an intervention in a single clinic or general practice (Corrigan *et al* , 2006) Box 7.3 contains an example.

Box 7.3   An example of qualitative study used to develop an intervention.

A qualitative study was undertaken by Henrickson *et al.* (2009) to develop and evaluate a pre-operative briefing – a short interaction structured by a checklist – for cardiovascular surgery. Focus groups were conducted with a range of surgical staff, and the findings used to help develop the briefing. The focus group findings indicated agreement among surgical staff concerning the benefits of briefings as well as their duration, location, content and potential barriers. The findings also indicated that staff did not, however, reach consensus on the timing of the brief or the roles and responsibilities of key participants.

Understanding processes

The second area in which qualitative methods can be used in evaluation is in exploring processes linked to the implementation of an intervention (Oakley *et al.*, 2006). Process-based evaluations focus on exploring how and why something happens during the development and/or implementation of an intervention rather than the results or impact obtained. In this context, qualitative methods allow detailed exploration of a range of issues, including how an intervention process or mechanism unfolds in the real world, the perceptions and contributions of different participants, whether an intervention is being implemented as intended and, if not, how it differs from what was planned and whether the intervention affects different groups in different ways (Lewin *et al.*, 2009a). An example of the use of qualitative approaches to explore processes linked to the implementation of an intervention is offered in Box 7.4.

Box 7.4   A qualitative study of intervention implementation processes.

Paquette-Warren *et al.* (2006) studied the implementation of a shared care mental health and nutrition primary care programme in Canada. Shared care is a model of integrated delivery in which practitioners from different disciplines, or with varied skills sets, collaborate to deliver appropriate care. The programme aimed to increase accessibility to high quality mental health and nutrition services in primary care. A qualitative evaluation was undertaken to obtain an understanding of the perceptions and experiences of the providers collaborating in this programme. Focus group discussions were conducted and content analysis used to explore the data obtained. The findings highlighted a number of strengths of the programme, including flexibility, improved communication, access to patient information, care continuity and provider and client satisfaction. The study concluded that, while there were challenges and variability among practices, the programme was viewed as providing better patient care overall.

Outcomes and impacts

Qualitative evaluation can be employed to identify the outcomes and impacts associated with an intervention. However, while the use of qualitative approaches for outcome evaluation is controversial (e.g. Kelly, 2004), such evaluations can be useful in three areas. First, qualitative data can be sed to explore the effects of a programme on outcomes that are difficult to measure quantitatively, such as the effects of teamwork interventions on morale and performance. Second, qualitative approaches can be used to explore whether an intervention is sustained over time. For example, focus group discussions with teams running primary health care centres could be used to assess whether efforts to improve information sharing between professionals were being sustained and whether these efforts were perceived as continuing to have benefits for providers and clients. Third, they can also be used to examine effects across different groups or sites, such as different wards within a hospital or primary health care centres in a local setting. Qualitative data may be useful in explaining why a teamwork intervention is effective in some and less effective in others.

Theory building and use of existing theory

Qualitative approaches may be used to build theory, for example, in developing models to explain teamwork phenomena (e.g., team communication, team collaboration, interprofessional learning). Conversely, theory can contribute to evaluation by providing a framework for approaching an issue or problem and can influence the collection, analysis and interpretation of data.

Theory may be useful in locating the findings within a broader (explanatory) framework. For example, in Regan de Bere's (2003) paper, draws upon Foucauldian theory to evaluate an interprofessional team course for physicians, nurses, social workers and service users based in mental health settings. She reports that before the initiative was delivered, participants held a range of different discourses. Specifically, they were able to draw simultaneously on both personal and professional discourses, as these tended to complement each other. Data gathered directly after the course indicated that the discourses held by the various practitioners had begun to merge to form a more 'generic collaborative discourse' (p. 119) that stressed an appreciation of different professional roles, respect for other professional groups and a support of teamwork.

Theory may also be useful in comparing the findings across studies. In addition, it can provide an approach to explaining why interventions succeed or fail, for example through suggesting underlying mechanisms of action (May *et al.*, 2007; Elwyn *et al.*, 2008).

Participation in evaluation

Participation of patients is increasingly seen to be important in health and social service provision. Initiatives like expert patient programmes (e.g. UK Expert Patients Programme, 2009) and collaborative patient-centred approaches (Health Canada, 2009) are examples. It has been suggested that this focus on participation has been important in promoting the use of qualitative approaches in evaluation (Murphy *et al.*, 1998). Participatory research methods – such as action research studies (see Box 6.3) – go further by attempting to involve stakeholders (e.g. members of an interprofessional team) in the research process itself. This may include framing the evaluation questions, interpreting the findings and sometimes involvement in data collection activities. This approach emerged from feminist critiques of research which highlighted power imbalances between the researchers and those who are 'researched' (Oakley, 1981), and indicated the need for a model that was less disempowering for research participants.

Participatory approaches have a number of advantages. For example, these methods build the commitment of stakeholders to the evaluation process and can provide additional insights regarding the evaluation question through more in-depth and trusting researcher–participant relations. A number of disadvantages to the approach have also been noted. These include the amount of time needed, difficulty in achieving high levels of participation, and assumptions that different stakeholders will be in agreement and able to work with each other in the research process. Participatory evaluation may also be seen as less 'neutral'. Furthermore, tension may be created if findings do not match stakeholders' expectations.

Limitations

Qualitative studies also have a number of limitations (Murphy *et al.*, 1998). First, causality – the extent to which any intervention effects identified in qualitative work can be attributed to the intervention is difficult to establish. Second, qualitative evaluators are often faced with the task of explaining and justifying their methodological approach to those not familiar with this type of work like health service managers. Third, a main critique of qualitative evaluations, generated from the positivist paradigm, concerns generalisability. This critique raises questions regarding the extent to which qualitative findings are applicable in contexts other than the one in which the research was undertaken (Green, 1999). Responding to this critique, Brewer (2000, p. 77) argues that, in qualitative research, 'generalisation involves theoretical inference from data to develop concepts and connections'. Such 'explanatory propositions' (Brewer, 2000, p. 151), it is suggested, may indicate ways in which study findings may explain similar behaviours, cases or events in other settings.

The use of mixed methods evaluation can overcome some of the limitations of qualitative studies, as we discuss below.

Mixed methods evaluations

Reliance on a single quantitative or qualitative method inevitably restricts the types of data that can be gathered and the insights that can be inferred from them. In mixed methods evaluation, different data collection approaches (e.g. documentary analysis, observations, interviews, surveys) are used at different points of time and for different purposes. These can provide more detailed understanding of the processes and outcomes associated with a particular intervention such as teamwork. Triangulation between quantitative and qualitative data can help generate a more comprehensive set of findings, as corroboration of ideas from one approach to another can occur (Rallis and Rossman, 2003). The use of mixed methods evaluation can also address a wider range of evaluation questions – including why, what, how and when – as different methods are best suited to different research questions. Another advantage is that differences between findings from different methods can be used to generate hypotheses and to identify areas requiring further investigation. Finally, mixed methods evaluation can help meet demands from commissioning agencies for comprehensive evaluations (e.g. O'Cathain *et al.*, 2007).

Mixed methods studies are becoming increasingly common in the research literature (see Box 7.5 for an example).

Box 7.5   A mixed methods study.

Cooper *et al.* (2007a, 2007b) describe a mixed methods study they undertook in a large UK-based ambulance service. The study aimed to identify factors affecting collaboration and to produce a model of collaborative practice. Collaboration was assessed using a range of approaches: direct observational ratings of communication skills, teamwork and leadership with emergency care practitioners; interviews with these practitioners and other stakeholders; and patient audit. The study indicated that practitioners' links with other professions were influenced by the specific roles of emergency care practitioners; factors related to education and training; and cultural perspectives, including power conflicts. Quantitative observational ratings showed that the higher the leadership rating of a practitioner, the greater the communication ability and teamworking. The authors concluded that the collaborative performance of emergency practitioners is variable, but that their role did seem to have an impact on teamwork, collaborative practices and patient care.

A range of typologies of mixed method designs have been proposed. The works of Greene and Caracelli (1997) and Tashakkori and Teddlie (2003), for example, provide useful overviews of how different methods can be used at different stages of a mixed methods study.

Underlying debates

Mixing qualitative and quantitative approaches does raise some important epistemological issues, as these approaches are rooted in different understandings of the social world. Some evaluators have taken a 'purist' approach to these debates, suggesting that it is not useful or sensible to mix paradigms within a single study as they represent fundamentally contrasting ways of knowing the world (e.g. Greene and Caracelli, 1997). Further, mixing methods may result in oversights of one method, thus undermining the quality of evaluations (O'Cathain *et al.*, 2008). Evaluators, however, more often take a 'pragmatic' approach, which acknowledges philosophical differences between paradigms but suggests that practical considerations are more important. These considerations include the complexity of interventions and contexts which, in turn, requires a range of methods; the need to use methods that are appropriate to a particular setting; and also the need to address multiple research questions within limited resources (Greene and Caracelli, 1997).

Of course, to some extent the divide between qualitative and quantitative methods is artificial. Rather, research approaches can be seen as a continuum between positivist (quantitative) and interpretivist (qualitative) approaches. It is also worth noting that methods, as procedures for gathering or analysing data, are not intrinsically linked to any particular paradigm.

Limitations

Limitations of mixed methods evaluation include difficulties regarding *how* to combine the findings of these different components, so that the whole is greater than the sum of the parts. In addition, using several different methods requires high levels of expertise within the evaluation team and this, in turn, may increase costs. Indeed, implementing mixed methods evaluations can be very resource intensive.

Conclusions and implications

Careful evaluation of interprofessional teamwork is needed to understand its nature, to advance our knowledge of this field and to identify the effects of teamwork on professionals and patients. Traditionally, however, interprofessional teamwork has been evaluated in an uncritical manner, typically relying on locally developed surveys or interview data with various team members. These approaches have tended to provide a normative view of teamworking rather than one grounded in data drawn from observation of teamworking in practice. Similarly, reviews of interprofessional teamwork also tend to be descriptive, rather than analytical. We have therefore attempted to present a more thoughtful approach to evaluation – an approach which is mindful of the complexity of teamwork and assesses the purpose (formative, summative), the intervention targets (inputs, processes, outcomes, impacts) as well the types of evidence (local, generalisable). We also outlined the comparative strengths and limitations of the quantitative, qualitative and mixed methods approaches that might be employed in a teamwork evaluation.

Thinking about the future, we see a key role for qualitative evaluation in generating, through careful observation, a better understanding of the nature of interprofessional team relations (for example, how unequal power relations between team members affect teamwork) and greater insight into the processes of change associated with interventions to promote teamwork. Through synthesis approaches such as meta-ethnography (e.g. Britten *et al.*, 2002; Barnett-Page and Thomas, 2009), qualitative approaches can also provide a firmer theoretical basis for interprofessional teamwork. Evaluation of interprofessional interactions could also be strengthened by the more rigorous use of quantitative methods, particularly randomised approaches to the assessment of the effects of teamwork interventions. In addition, mixed methods approaches, evaluation of the sustainability of teamwork interventions over time and more thoughtful use of review work to better understand, and build on, existing research evidence are important.

8 Synthesising studies of interprofessional teamwork

Introduction

The previous three chapters have explored and critiqued how different teamwork interventions may be designed and implemented, informed by theory and evaluated. In this chapter we build on these discussions by presenting a synthesis of three studies of interprofessional teamwork which we have undertaken during the past 15 years. The studies were based in three countries: South Africa, the UK and Canada. Our aim in presenting this synthesis is to provide an insight into how we designed and evaluated a number of different interprofessional interventions and also discuss our experiences related to this work.

Initially we provide the contextual information related to each of the studies before presenting details on the methodological process related to how we analysed and synthesised these data sets. Findings from this synthesis are then presented in terms of the main themes from across the three studies; the aim is to offer an in-depth empirical account of how interprofessional collaboration and teamwork operate in these different clinical contexts. Lastly, we discuss the broader implications of this work in relation to other settings.

Background context

The contextual information is presented below, including the local clinical and institutional settings of the studies. This provides a frame for understanding local processes and findings particularly in respect to how each site evolved from design to implementation and evaluation.

Study 1: South Africa

This study emerged from early clinical audit work on general medicine wards based in a large teaching hospital in Cape Town, which suggested that professionals worked in a routinised manner and were not responsive to individual patient needs. As a result, senior clinicians collaborated with researchers and clinical managers to develop LOCIS (Level of Care Intervention Study) – an intervention which aimed to tailor the level of care provided to each patient according to need. This tailoring required an improvement in interprofessional communication among all ward staff, especially between nursing and medicine staff. The intervention aimed at improving interprofessional relationships and also the delivery of care.

LOCIS included four elements. First, team-building activities designed to improve interprofessional relations were provided to ward staff in order to clarify each profession's contribution, responsibilities and frustrations. These team-building activities also aimed to promote agreement on shared patient care values and goals, and to ensure that staff would meet as named individuals rather than as members of separate professions. Second, a reorganisation of staff occurred in which nursing and medical staff were split into two teams, each consisting of one senior physician, a number of junior physicians and nurses in order to provide better targeted and more responsive care. Third, nursing staff were mandated by their clinical leaders to eliminate task-oriented nursing (which focused on task completion rather than being responsive to patient needs) and to share knowledge and patient responsibility among all members of the nursing team. Fourth, each medical–nursing team was mandated by their clinical leaders to conduct a daily joint planning ward round, during which care plans were reviewed for each patient and signed by both nurse and physician.

LOCIS employed a controlled-before-and-after design to evaluate its processes and impact. Quantitative and qualitative data were collected in the form of patient care processes, outcome and satisfaction measures, staff surveys, observations and interviews with a range of junior and senior clinical staff.

For further information about this study, see Zwarenstein *et al.* (2003).

Study 2: The UK

Based in a large teaching hospital in London, this study was undertaken in a medical directorate consisting of five general medical wards and one emergency admissions ward. An intervention was designed to respond to concerns within the medical directorate that the distribution of medical teams (including senior and junior physicians) and their patients across a large number of medical wards had a range of negative effects including:

- Lengthy ward rounds
- Difficulties for medical teams in getting to know ward-based teams, which included nurses, therapists, social workers and pharmacists. This, it was thought, resulted in less involvement by ward-based staff (e.g. nurses, therapists) in decision-making on patient care
- Inefficiencies due to medical staff having to move between wards
- Patients not always receiving optimal care if they were admitted, within the rota system, to a physician from a speciality different to that of their initial presenting condition.

To address these concerns, a ward-based medical team (WBMT) system was developed and introduced by the directorate leaders and clinicians. This system aimed to promote effective collaboration by basing each medical team and the patients for whom they were caring on one 'home' ward, rather than across multiple wards. A new triage system was also introduced to ensure that patients were managed by the appropriate specialists. As part of this, a list of health conditions was identified that would require the transfer of the patient to a medical team focusing on a particular speciality.

The study aimed to explore the impact of the WBMT system on interprofessional collaboration and on the clinical service delivered to patients. A mixed methods research design was used to develop a comprehensive understanding of the effects of the new system. Questionnaire, audit, observational, interview and documentary data were collected with practitioners, managers and patients before introduction of the WBMT system and also 1 month and then 9 months after its introduction.

For further information about this study, see Reeves and Lewin *et al.* (2003) and Reeves and Lewin (2004).

Study 3: Canada

The SCRIPT (Structuring Communication Relationships for Interprofessional Teamwork) programme was a multi-year project. It had one broad aim – to work with staff to introduce interprofessional education and collaboration within a number of local medical, primary and rehabilitation care teaching units and practice settings. To achieve this aim, the project had three key objectives: to design empirically based interventions to foster interprofessional collaboration and teamwork; to pilot-test interventions; and, if successful, to implement these across the three selected clinical contexts. A multi-method study was designed by a team of researchers and clinicians to explore factors that facilitated or impeded interprofessional communication across these clinical contexts in Toronto.

Within the general medicine arm of this study, a series of observations and interviews were undertaken to understand the nature of interprofessional teamwork within this setting. As a result, researchers developed the following four-step communication intervention designed to be employed by professionals in their face-to-face interprofessional collaboration:

1. Introduce oneself to the member(s) of the other profession by name
2. State to the other individual(s) one's own professional role in the team and describe it with respect to the patient under discussion
3. Share with the other professional their unique, profession-specific issues, problems or plans relating to the patient
4. Elicit feedback from the other professional by using prompts such as 'Do you have any concerns?' or 'Is there something else I should consider?'

These four steps were based upon the following two assumptions: first, if professionals continuously introduced themselves by name and role, any confusion

Table 8.1 Overview of the key features of the included interprofessional studies.

	Study 1: LOCIS	Study 2: WBMT	Study 3: SCRIPT
Setting	Cape Town, South Africa	London, United Kingdom	Toronto, Canada
Intervention(s)	Package of interventions including organisational change, training in teamworking and daily joint planning ward rounds between nurses and doctors	Ward-based medical teams to enhance the quality of interprofessional interactions and teamwork	A communication protocol to enhance interprofessional communication among general medicine staff
Intervention focus	Organisational and relational	Organisational	Relational
Overall research design	Controlled before-and-after study	Descriptive longitudinal study	Planned as RCT but this was found not to be feasible. Descriptive study conducted
Evaluation methods	Mixed methods	Mixed methods	Mixed methods

or anonymity would be reduced. Second, if professionals shared their perspective and elicited a collegial point of view, opportunities to solve a patient care problem would be enhanced. Strauss's (1978) theory of negotiated order underpinned the design of the intervention (see Chapter 5). Evaluation of SCRIPT was planned as a randomised control trials (RCT) with an in-depth process evaluation across five hospitals, involving 20 general medicine units.

For more information about this study, see Zwarenstein *et al.* (2007), Miller *et al.* (2008), Gotlib Conn *et al.* (2009) and Reeves *et al.* (2009c).

Table 8.1 provides an overview of information from these three interprofessional cases.

Study selection

Applying our interprofessional typology of in Chapter 3, these three studies can be seen as examples of 'teamwork' within a continuum of other forms of interprofessional work (see Figure 3.1). However, we would see their place as near to the boundary with 'collaboration'. This is because the interactions we described below contains both elements of teamwork (including shared responsibility for decisions and activities, interdependence and team tasks which were often complex) and some elements of collaboration (in that team tasks were fairly predictable and not very urgent and a shared identity was not a strong feature of these teams). Without claiming that they were exemplars of teamworking, these studies do provide a rich data set for understanding issues related to the nature of interprofessional relations in acute general medicine settings. Such settings are the site for a large proportion of interprofessional care delivered within health systems across a range of jurisdictions.

Analysis and synthesis

While all three studies gathered both quantitative and qualitative data, this chapter reports a synthesis of the following qualitative data:

- Over 200 hours of observations and 30 interviews with a range of different junior and senior health care professionals (South Africa)
- 90 hours of observations and 74 interviews with a range of different junior and senior health care professionals (UK)
- 155 hours of observations, 53 interviews with a range of different junior and senior health care professionals, and 5 hours of work-shadowing data from a range of ward-based professionals (Canada).

We focus on the qualitative data sets – the observations in particular – as they provide a rich detailed account of the nature of interprofessional relations 'in action'. As we noted in Chapter 6, the current teamwork literature tends to rely on individuals' *perceptions* of teamwork which can only provide a normative account of team relations, not an actual insight into the realities of teamwork.

The following process was undertaken to analyse and synthesise materials for this chapter. Drawing on elements of the meta-ethnographic approach (Noblit and Hare, 1988), which aims to translate ideas and concepts across different studies, we first read and re-read each of the reports generated from the three studies, noting their key themes and any explanations offered. Second, we abstracted information from each study on its aims, settings, theoretical background, sampling, data collection and data-analysis approaches, findings in the form of key themes and any recommendations offered on interprofessional working. For each study, abstraction was completed by one of us who had not been involved in the study and then discussed with the others. Third, we compared and contrasted the key themes to identify related concepts, which in turn were the basis for the synthesis we present below.

Key themes

We now offer key themes from our synthesis. We initially outline the nature of interprofessional teamwork in the study settings prior to the implementation of the interventions. We then go on to outline how the interventions affected (or failed to affect) the nature of interprofessional relations across these settings. Table 8.2 provides an overview of key findings.

Table 8.2   Main findings from the three studies.

Study 1: LOCIS – South Africa	Study 2: WBMT – The UK	Study 3: SCRIPT – Canada
Key findings – pre-intervention		
Most IP interactions were terse and serendipitous. Those involving physicians were medically led and were in the form of 'orders'.	Typically, IP interactions were brief and serendipitous. Those involving physicians were generally medically led and were in the form of 'requests'.	In general, IP interactions were terse and serendipitous. Those involving physicians were medically led using 'orders'.
Intraprofessional and IP interactions (involving nurses, therapists and pharmacists) were lengthier and friendlier.	Physician–nurse relations slightly more cordial than the other two sites.	Intraprofessional and IP interactions lengthier and friendlier.
Weekly team meetings physician-dominated.	Intraprofessional and other IP interactions were lengthier and generally friendly.	Daily team meetings had cordial interactions, though provided limited IP communication.
	Weekly team meetings provided a regular forum for communication. Poor attendance of physicians and nurses (due to competing commitments) often undermined their value.	
Key findings – post-intervention		
Improved IP working with professionals more aware of communication.	Physicians' interactions with other professionals were more regular. Consequently, nurses and other staff felt there was a better IP rapport.	IP interactions and nature of relations remained largely unchanged.
Physician–nurse interactions seen to have become less hierarchical.	IP interactions remained terse. Weekly IP team meetings remained poorly attended by physicians and nurses.	
Physicians displayed a greater awareness of the constraints on nurses' time.		

Note: IP = interprofessional.

Interprofessional interactions before intervention

General nature of interprofessional interactions

In general, the wards across all settings were very busy. At any one time, a number of people, including relatives and friends of the patients as well as staff from other units within the hospital, could be entering or leaving. Staff were also consulting with patients, undertaking ward rounds and minor procedures, completing paperwork, dealing with telephonic and verbal enquiries from other professionals, patients and relatives, arranging interventions for patients, cleaning the ward and making beds, serving food and drink, as well as attending to the care needs of patients. The following extract, taken from the UK study, indicates the nature of this setting:

> A senior physician comes into the ward and asks who is in charge. A junior nurse says, 'I am'. 'Oh', he replies, 'I would like to speak to a staff nurse'. He then talks to one of the staff nurses about the transport required by a patient who is going for a procedure outside of the hospital. [...] A junior physician comes into the ward and goes to the bedside of one of the patients. She then goes to fetch some syringes and goes back to the bedside to take blood specimens. She checks the specimens, tells a staff nurse that they can 'go up' [to the laboratory] and goes back into the patient bay. A few minutes later another junior physician comes into the ward, goes to the nurse' station and asks for urgent bloods to be collected. He then hangs about waiting for a call that will let him know where his ward round is. He then leaves the ward. At the same time, one of the staff nurses is trying to help a person who is looking for a relative who was moved from the admissions ward to another part of the hospital. A dietician comes to the nurses' station and asks this nurse some questions about a patient's eating. She makes a note in the folder and chats to the nurse about future care with regard to eating. (Observational data, UK)

Findings from observational data gathered in the Canadian and South African settings provided very similar insights regarding the nature of interprofessional interactions in these settings. Indeed, our observations indicated that interprofessional interactions, especially those involving physicians, across the three sites were generally short, largely unstructured and often serendipitous. If a professional had a query, they would usually look around the ward for another professional who might be able to answer it. If the appropriate professional was found, the two might have a brief discussion and then continue with their other tasks.

Interactions between physicians and other professionals on the wards

Across the three sites, we found that interprofessional interactions which involved physicians and other health and social care professionals (e.g. nurses, therapists and social workers) were particularly terse, as illustrated in the following extracts:

> The sister [senior nurse] asked the intern [junior physician] when they were going to do the rounds and he answered that he was waiting for the registrar [...], noting that 'we will call you'. (Observational data, South Africa)

> An intern comes in and grabs three charts from the cart. He asks the social worker if any forms need to be filled out for a patient then leaves. (Observational data, Canada)

In general, interprofessional interactions appeared to be anonymous – few staff knew the names or roles and scopes of practice of their colleagues. Across the three sites, the data indicated that a significant proportion of interactions involving physicians were unidirectional rather than taking the form of a discussion. Typically, such interactions were from physician to nurse, as illustrated below:

> A house officer [junior physician] asks the charge nurse, who is busy with the task of wheeling a commode through the ward, for a dynamap machine. She tells him to ask the nurse on the other side of the ward. (Observational data, UK)

In the UK, these interactions were focused largely on providing medical 'requests' for the progression of care. This was also the case in Canada and South Africa, where this type of interaction was termed medical 'orders', perhaps reflecting the character of these interactions. Furthermore, nurses and therapists and other professionals offered input primarily when prompted by physicians. For example, while many physicians in the South African study perceived their communication with registered nurses to be satisfactory, their comments suggested that this view was based on nurses accepting their orders:

> Communication with the sisters is good. We all have responsibilities for the patients. As long as they carry out their orders I don't have a problem. (Physician interview, South Africa)

> We talk when we need to. I have no complaints. (Physician interview, South Africa)

In the UK, we found that nurses' communication with physicians was focused almost entirely on obtaining a medical response to questions they had about care. While physicians in the UK study were fairly responsive to these questions, those in Canada and South Africa often ignored nurses' questions or comments, or referred the nurses back to the original order or instruction that had been given. While not close, relations between physicians and nurses in the UK setting appeared slightly more cordial than in the other two settings.

In addition, across the sites, ward-based interactions between physicians and other professionals largely involved junior physicians. Indeed, there was a noticeable absence of senior physicians from the wards for most of the working day. As a result, most day-to-day interprofessional activities and decisions regarding patient care were taken by their juniors (registrars, residents, interns, house officers).

Interactions among professionals other than physicians on the wards

By contrast, data from the three study sites indicated far more interprofessional communication among professionals other than physicians on the wards. Interactions that involved nurses, therapists, pharmacists and social workers were generally friendlier and less rushed, as the following extracts indicate:

> The speech language pathologist and dietician are still talking. The speech language pathologist feels stressed [...] 'I need a psych consult,' she jokes. (Observational data, Canada)

> A nurse and a physiotherapist have a discussion about a patient – the physiotherapist explains problems she is having with a patient [...] the exchange lasts for a good ten minutes. I am struck by the depth and length of this discussion. (Observational data, UK)

As the extracts above indicate, these types of interactions often involved discussion of care issues and exchanges of a humorous nature.

Interprofessional meetings

Interprofessional meetings were held in all three settings with a range of purposes. In the Canadian setting, interprofessional rounds were held everyday. While interactions during these rounds were friendlier than on the wards, interprofessional discussion was still limited. In both the UK and Canada, nurses reported refraining from participating in or interrupting interprofessional meetings. This was in part because they found these meetings were of limited use to their work. Also, nurses sometimes felt intimidated by senior physicians or felt that their views were not valued. Nurses and other professionals therefore felt that their opinions went largely unvoiced during these meetings.

Physicians in these two settings often complained that interprofessional meetings were of little use and saw the main beneficiaries as being occupational therapists, physiotherapists and social workers:

> From the medical perspective, the information that is shared at [our interprofessional meetings] is not always useful, like what the functional ability of a patient is. (Physician interview, Canada)

In the UK, physicians and, to a lesser extent, nurses saw ward rounds as an important forum for interprofessional communication. In practice, though, they were generally a uniprofessional medical activity. Even if other professionals attended ward rounds, they tended to be on the periphery and therefore not involved in any of the clinical decision-making that occurred.

One regular mechanism for interprofessional communication and information exchange in the UK setting was the weekly interprofessional meeting. These gatherings were intended to allow physicians, nurses, occupational therapists, physiotherapists, social workers and care coordinators working with each medical team to update one another, discuss the progress and problems with patient care and plan patient discharges. Some professionals considered these meetings a key mechanism for interprofessional interaction:

> Those [interprofessional] meetings are really important. That's when we find out [. . .] the nitty gritty of what is actually wrong with them [patients]. (Social worker interview, UK)

However, both physicians and nurses regularly failed to attend interprofessional meetings, which often delayed decisions on patient care and discharge. Nurses cited heavy workloads combined with a shortage of staff as the reasons for their non-attendance. For the physicians, especially the senior ones, the nature of their duties meant that they were often working in other parts of the hospital or undertaking ward rounds or clinics during the time scheduled for these meetings.

In the South African setting, interprofessional meetings to discuss the social circumstances of patients were usually controlled by registrars and medical interns who often ignored differing views from other staff. Most information was provided by interns while registrars almost always gave orders regarding when patients had to be seen by a social worker or specialist nurse. The ward nurses seldom said or were asked anything.

Spatial factors

A mechanism employed by staff in both Canada and the UK to overcome interprofessional communication difficulties was the use of the hospital corridors for informal information exchange:

> We catch up on the corridor [. . .] informally speak to physios and OTs and social workers, so there is good group contact there. (Physician interview, UK)

While most patients in the UK site were in multi-bed wards, patients in the Canadian setting generally had private rooms. This decreased the likelihood of opportunistic interprofessional interaction at the bedside and increased the importance of hospital corridors for communication. By contrast, the use of such informal mechanisms was not reported to be used by the professionals in the South African study.

Uniprofessional relations

Across the three sites, uniprofessional interactions were richer than interprofessional discussions and included both work and social elements. In the Canadian setting, many professionals saw interprofessional rounds as a low priority and uniprofessional activities as more important. This was particularly so for physicians. As noted above, there were also more social interactions within professional groups than between them:

> A resident jokes that they will be answering pages only before the [hockey] game starts. Another resident explains that they will be watching [medical drama]. A third resident tells her it is a repeat, and when she asks which episode, two residents teasingly respond that, 'it's the one where someone gets an IV and is intubated, and then something else happens and then someone sleeps with someone.' There is a lot of laughter. (Observational data, Canada)

Many of the physicians in the UK setting saw collaboration as an activity involving different medical teams or specialities rather than other professional groups. For example, observations revealed significant discussion at management meetings in the clinical directorate on ways of improving collaboration between medical teams and with other medical specialties. By contrast, ways of improving interprofessional collaboration received far less attention.

Interprofessional interactions after intervention

Following the implementation of the respective interventions, in all three settings, nurse–physician relations remained central to interprofessional collaboration. In both Canada and the UK, the nature of communication between physicians and other professionals did not change significantly following the interventions – it remained terse, task-oriented and seldom included any social content:

> The charge nurse asks a passing physician, 'are you looking after patient X?' The physician says, 'no, X is'. The charge nurse then asks, 'What's his bleep [page] number?' The physician gives it and goes on. (Observational data, UK)

Although in the UK, due to the formation of WBMTs, interprofessional communication between the physicians and other professionals did become more frequent. By contrast, there appeared to be more interprofessional collaboration in the South African setting following the intervention. Through working together more closely on the ward level, professionals appeared to have become more aware of the need for better communication and saw this aspect of their work as having improved:

> The teams now involve everybody, doctors, colleagues, as well as pupil and student nurses. Even the domestics [domestic workers or cleaners]. Now I experience them as all behaving as part of a team. Five months ago it was not like that, but now I can see the difference. They are suddenly talking to each other. (Auxiliary staff, interview, South Africa)

There were a number of aspects to this change in interactions in South Africa – communication between physicians and nurses was seen to have become less hierarchical at ward level, medical staff displayed a greater awareness of the constraints on nurses' time, and both nurses and physicians described having a better understanding of each others' roles and those of their colleagues on the wards:

> This kind of understanding between nursing and medicine is improved by working in a specific team. I would feel free to tell Doctor A what I think. (Nurse interview, South Africa)

In South Africa, as a result of the intervention, both nurses and physicians also reported improved communication with patients during ward rounds and more generally:

> We are more involved with our patients than before. I spend more time talking to them, finding out about their domestic situation to enable me to plan discharge and I tend to give more information to them than in the past. (Nurse interview, South Africa)

In the UK, interviews with patients and professionals suggested that patients had somewhat better access to staff following the intervention, although they still encountered difficulty at times. The Canadian study did not include a patient perspective.

Across all three settings, following the implementation of the interventions, professionals continued to place very little 'social capital' (Bourdieu, 1986) on the use of communication as a mechanism for improving interprofessional relations and/or the delivery of care. Instead, they continued use communication for the completion of their profession-specific tasks. Physicians in particular, often did not see any benefit to this communication and, consequently, it became invisible to them. For example, physicians in the Canadian study described interprofessional meetings as a largely 'redundant' part of their work. In both the UK and Canada, there were numerous examples of physicians continuing to ignore or not respond to other professionals when working on the wards:

> Two senior-looking physicians come into the ward. One starts using the computer at the nurses' station – almost pushing a health care assistant out of the way – while the other reads a newspaper that is lying on the desk in the nurses' station. They don't speak to the health care assistant who is sitting at the nurses' station, but talk to each other about some problem with the computer. (Observational data, UK)

Linked to this, there continued to be very little social communication on these wards. This may be because these professionals saw no value in maintaining communication, whose only perceived value is social, despite the importance of such forms of interaction in maintaining relations with other professionals.

As indicated above, only two of the interventions (South Africa and the UK) resulted in marginal gains for interprofessional teamwork. While the South Africa study reported most improvements, with increases in the frequency and quality of interactions with physicians (though no change in the underlying nature of relations); data from the Canadian study indicated that the intervention had no detectable effect. The longevity of these interventions was also limited. For example, in South Africa, despite some changes in nurse–physician relations, senior management decided not to undertake any further implementation across the hospital. Similarly, in the UK setting, despite some gains, the intervention was not implemented any further. In addition, attempts to obtain funding at this site to expand the intervention to include a team-building element were unsuccessful. In Canada, due to limited physician support and the absence of a local champion, following completion of a pilot-testing phase there was no further intervention activity. Plans for a multi-hospital RCT therefore became unfeasible.

Discussion

The three studies reported in this chapter are accounts of teamwork 'in action', based on detailed qualitative analysis of a substantial body of ethnographic observations of interprofessional teamwork and collaboration. As noted above, while most analyses draw on individuals' perceptions of teamwork, and are therefore often normative in nature, these data provide rare empirical insights into how teamwork is undertaken in practice. For example, this approach has helped to highlight the use of informal modes of communication, such as corridor conversations, alongside more formal teamworking activities, such as interprofessional meetings.

The data are also unusual in that they are drawn from a similar level of the health system (general medicine wards within large, tertiary referral hospitals based in urban locations) but from very different socio-economic and political settings (Canada, South Africa and the UK). Important differences between the settings include the level of autonomy of physicians, which due to remuneration arrangements is higher in Canada compared to the other two sites, and demographic characteristics of patients, with most patients in the South African study being black and of low socio-economic status; those in the UK setting being very ethnically diverse but generally of low socio-economic status; and those in Canada being largely elderly and of higher socio-economic status.

Juxtaposition of these three cases is useful in highlighting both aspects of teamworking that seem to be consistent across country settings (e.g. terse interactions) as well as elements that differ (e.g. contrasting local contexts), thereby helping to tease out the 'core' features of teamworking in acute medicine settings. Importantly, differences across the study settings in the socio-economic status of patients did not seem to have an impact on the nature of interprofessional collaboration.

While not included here, data on patient perspectives from South Africa and the UK were useful in understanding the impacts of the interventions on patient experiences of care (e.g. Reeves and Lewin *et al.*, 2003). For example, patients and their families in the UK reported having better access to physicians following implementation of the WBMT intervention, which made it easier for them to obtain information and plan for care following discharge. (As noted above, the Canadian study did not include a patient perspective).

The interventions in both South Africa and the UK did not explicitly draw upon theory in their development – both were designed in a pragmatic manner to help resolve identified difficulties in the provision of care within these settings. By contrast, the SCRIPT intervention drew on Strauss's (1978) negotiated order perspective to design the four-step communication activity, which helped developed an approach which was sensitive to the nature and role of negotiation within a general medicine context.

Factors affecting the uptake of the interventions in the different settings

As we discussed above, the uptake of the interventions, and their consequent impacts on interprofessional teamworking was stronger in the South African and UK cases, compared to the Canadian case. Box 8.1 outlines three factors which affected the uptake of the interventions in these different settings.

As Box 8.1 indicates, the general absence of interprofessional champions, wider professional/organisational support and role modelling can diminish the impact of the interprofessional teamwork interventions. Furthermore, differences between physician autonomy and status within Canada compared with the other two settings added an additional factor which compounded the others and impeded any improvement in teamwork associated with this intervention.

> **Box 8.1**   Factors which limited the effects of teamwork interventions.
>
> *Local champions.* There was both buy-in and championing of the intervention by key senior staff in South Africa and the UK, particularly by lead physicians. This was not the case in the Canadian setting. As a consequence of the work of local champions, senior-level physicians and nurses in the participating facilities in South Africa and the UK either gave instructions to their junior staff, or achieved their support for the changes entailed by the intervention. Furthermore, organisational changes needed to support the intervention were made by senior levels of management.
>
> *Ward-level role modelling.* In all three settings, there was a general absence of senior physicians from the wards for most of the working day. Most day-to-day decisions regarding patient care were taken by registrars (residents), particularly in Canada and the UK. Consequently, there were few opportunities for senior physicians to 'role model' more effective forms of teamworking to their junior staff.
>
> *Autonomy and status of physicians.* In both the UK and South Africa, physicians work within publicly funded hospitals, and appear to have lower levels of autonomy than in Canada. This appears to be linked to the fact that, in Canada, physicians are effectively self-employed, while in South Africa and the UK they are salaried employees. As a result, physicians in these two settings appeared to have a greater attachment and commitment to building effective teams.

Implications for teamwork

A number of cross-cutting implications for the evaluation of teamworking emerged from the three studies. First, a striking outcome from this synthesis was the commonalities underlying team performance in the three settings. Further comparative work, drawing on data from hospitals in other settings, would be valuable in exploring the extent to which these findings are generalisable on a wider basis. In particular, work is needed on settings that have been influenced less strongly by the publicly funded systems of care such as the UK, Canada and South Africa; on hospitals in low-income country settings; and on non-academic hospitals. Work is therefore needed to explore the generalisability of these findings, and their implications, to teams in other health care settings, such as primary care teams, stroke care teams and operating-room teams.

Second, as we noted above, the South African intervention, which employed a multifaceted approach – interprofessional education (to learn the principles of teamwork and increase their understanding other professionals' roles/responsibilities) as well as other interventions such as a reorganisation in the delivery of care – appeared to have more impact than the UK and Canadian sites which both employed a single intervention.

In addition, given the imbalanced historical foundations from which the health and social care professions emerged, interventions aimed at improving communication and teamworking must take account of the social inequalities that exist between physicians and other professionals. Furthermore, future interventions need to be implemented with rigorous evaluation, preferably in the form of a mixed method approach – an RCT with an in-depth, parallel qualitative evaluation to explore the barriers and facilitators to implementing teamwork interventions. Such work needs to be undertaken across a number of different team contexts such as surgery, day care units and stroke units to widen our understanding of how teams function in these settings.

Finally, the types of interventions that may be useful in improving interprofessional teamworking in hospital wards remain unclear – gains reported in the South African study may not be applicable in all settings. Indeed, due to issues of heterogeneity between interventions and context, it can be difficult to draw generalisable inferences about elements of effectiveness for interprofessional interventions (Zwarenstein *et al.*, 2009).

Ideas for the future

Based on our synthesis, Box 8.2 offers a series of implications for the future design of interventions to improve interprofessional teamworking.

As Box 8.2 illustrates, there are a number of important conceptual, empirical and theoretical issues which need to be considered in the design of interventions which aim to improve interprofessional teamworking.

Conclusions

In this chapter we presented a synthesis of three studies which evaluated the nature of teamwork interventions within general medical settings across three countries. We found a number of significant similarities in the nature of interprofessional collaboration across the three contrasting settings. Our synthesis also revealed that achieving improvement in teamwork and communication on hospital wards can be complex, as a number of factors need to be in place for this, including the need for interprofessional champions, committed leadership, support from professional groups (medicine, in particular) as well as from senior management. Methodologically, the use of an in-depth qualitative approach which gathers both observation *and* interviews can provide important insights into why such interventions may fail or succeed. We also discussed the use of theory in developing interventions to help understand the nature of existing forms of interprofessional teamwork is needed. In addition, we argued that the generalisability of the

Box 8.2   Implications for the future design of teamwork interventions.

- There are multiple factors affecting, and constraints to, achieving change in interprofessional teamworking in acute care and other settings. The complexity of the underlying problem means that an in-depth understanding of teamwork and local context issues is vital for the design and implementation of interventions.
- Constraints to teamwork, such as temporal–spatial limitations, may be difficult to overcome. Nonetheless, potential gains for patients and professionals are likely to be high from interventions that aim to address these factors.
- Substantial input from senior stakeholders, in particular medicine, is needed to take forward any intervention which aims to improve teamwork.
- Greater access by junior staff to senior medical staff could both provide a mechanism for role modelling interprofessional activities and increase the pace of medical decision-making in general medical contexts.
- Frequent organisational restructuring, as well as the constant barrage of other policy changes and shifting priorities, has the potential to divert management attention away from attempts to facilitate improved interprofessional teamwork. The same is true at the professional level. It is likely that only a sustained focus on interprofessional teamwork will achieve lasting improvements for collaboration, patient care and outcomes.
- The design of interventions to promote interprofessional teamworking should be facilitated through the explicit use of theory. Currently, much of the literature, including that describing intervention design, does not draw on theory in an explicit manner. This continues to hinder the development in the field.
- The use of research methods such as ethnography can provide an in-depth account of the nature of interprofessional teamwork. As such, their use should be encouraged to help design and develop teamwork interventions.
- Interprofessional teamwork interventions are complex. Their design may also be facilitated through the process outlined in the recently updated UK Medical Research Council framework for the development and evaluation of complex interventions (see Appendix 1).
- Further longitudinal research would be useful to assess the longer-term impact of interventions to promote interprofessional teamworking.

findings from this synthesis to other general medicine wards is good, particularly as findings were very similar across three quite different settings. There is less certainty, however, that these findings can be generalised to other clinical contexts such as operating-room teams, diabetes teams or stroke teams, given the different nature of how teamwork may operate in these settings.

9 Ways forward

Introduction

In this chapter we draw together the narrative threads of the book. In doing so, we initially offer a reflection and summary of key issues we have previously discussed. We then present our teamwork leaders' views for the future of interprofessional teamwork before offering our own ideas in relation to enhancing the design and implementation of interventions to improve teamwork. We also present some ideas on how to strengthen the evidence base for interprofessional teamwork.

Reflection and summary

First, we briefly revisit, summarise and reflect upon the contents of the preceding eight chapters in which we explored, discussed and critiqued a range of dimensions related to interprofessional teamwork.

In Chapter 1, we outlined some of the 'basics' of interprofessional teamwork to help understand how it is commonly understood as well as why teamwork is regarded as a central approach for helping to address a range of health and social care delivery problems. We also traced the emergence of a number of interprofessional teamwork initiatives which had occurred in a variety of countries. Finally, we offered some direct experiences of interprofessional teamwork from a number of different professionals based in different clinical settings.

In Chapter 2 we outlined a range of important political, social and economic developments which have emerged in the past decade that have, collectively, created a demand for interprofessional teamwork. Indeed, developments such as the patient safety initiative, the move towards collaborative patient-centred care as well as wider changes like the shift towards chronic illnesses can be regarded as key *drivers* which have contributed to the growing amount of teamwork activities that have been witnessed across the world.

We next explored, in Chapter 3, a range of key concepts and issues related to interprofessional teamwork to understand its conceptual foundations. We reviewed and critiqued a number of different team definitions, typologies and factors which affect team performance. We also introduced our notion of *team tasks* and discussed how predictability, urgency and complexity can affect interprofessional teamwork in important ways. In addition, we presented our *typology of interprofessional work* – teamwork, collaboration, coordination, networking – and discussed our *contingency approach* to reflect the different types of interprofessional work that can occur in different settings such as operating rooms, general medical wards and primary care clinics. We also introduced our notion of an *adaptive interprofessional team* – a team who can shift from one type of interprofessional work depending upon the needs of their patients. Finally, we problematised the use of teamwork approaches developed in the airline, quality and sports industries which have been gaining popularity in health and social care settings.

In Chapter 4 we presented our interprofessional framework in which we synthesised a range of teamwork factors into four domains: relational, processual, organisational and contextual. Through this discussion we explored how different factors such as professional power, hierarchy, gender, culture, team processes and organisational support affected interprofessional teamwork in different ways. We also discussed how these factors can affect teamwork individually and collectively.

In Chapter 5 we drew upon a range of social science theories to deepen our understanding of interprofessional teamwork and its potential role in the development and evaluation of teamwork interventions. We framed our discussion in this chapter by use of our four teamwork domains to show how different micro, mid-range and macro theories can yield different insights and understanding in the nature of interprofessional teamwork.

We explored, in Chapter 6, how different relational, processual, organisational and contextual interventions have been developed to improve interprofessional teamwork in a number of different ways. We also discussed the role of single and multifaceted interventions and how limitations in intervention design (e.g. a lack of critical analysis) can undermine the ability of interventions to achieve meaningful and lasting changes in the way interprofessional teams work together.

In Chapter 7 we argued that careful evaluation of interprofessional teamwork is needed in order to assist providers, policy makers and managers in their efforts to improve teamwork as well as advance our knowledge of the field. We also noted how most empirical accounts of interprofessional teamwork have been undertaken in an uncritical manner. We then went on to discuss why more thoughtful evaluation is needed to take into account the complexities of teamwork by use of qualitative, quantitative and mixed methods approaches.

In Chapter 8 we presented a synthesis of three studies based in Canada, South Africa and the UK to provide an account of our work designing and evaluating different interprofessional interventions. Our synthesis revealed that achieving improvement in teamwork and communication in acute settings in different contexts is a *very* complex process, involving a wide range of logistic, organisational and professional factors. We also outlined the need for theory in the design of interventions and how the use of ethnographic data can yield some important insights into why such interventions may succeed or fail.

Underpinning our exploration and discussion of the varying issues related to interprofessional teamwork were our various standpoints, which focused on being:

- Critical – to provide a text that could probe current assumptions, arguments and evidence related to interprofessional teamwork
- Pluralistic – to employ an approach which values contrasting views and understandings of teamwork
- Pragmatic – to keep thinking tied to the real world in order to provide a realistic account of the nature of teamwork and its impact
- Reflexive – to be thoughtful about our own work, views and experiences of teamwork when discussing it with others
- Optimistic – despite the multitude of challenges we have discussed in the book, to remain optimistic about the future of teamwork.

We incorporated these approaches to attempt to provide a different (missing) perspective on teamwork – one which problematised teamwork and also employed some new angles to think about an activity which, as we noted at the start of the book, has now become ingrained and largely accepted as a normal part of the health and social care landscape.

Some perspectives for the future of teamwork

In Chapter 2, we provided the perspectives of teamwork leaders on the current *gaps* in our understanding of interprofessional teamwork. We now go back to the leaders for their ideas for the future of teamwork in terms of what work needs to be undertaken to advance our knowledge in this area.

A view from Canada:

In both the post-secondary education system and health care system, organised surveys need to assess the curricula across human health services programs. They need to know how much time, effort, energy and money is invested in teamwork. They need to look at their capacity and willingness to train students and workers as team members. They need to ask: do they have this capacity, what does the training look like? How is it funded? Where does the funding come from, and what are the policies that drive funds to be allocated to teamwork development? (Teamwork leader 1, Canada)

Practitioners need to be provided with the time to explore the dimensions of unidisciplinary learning and how this impacts on their ability to work collaboratively. They need to learn to articulate their own roles, knowledge and skills to their colleagues in other disciplines. All team members need to learn to value the knowledge and skills that each member brings to the team and where each has unique and shared areas. They need to develop the means to jointly assess patients and to be respectful in the data they collect from patients and their relatives. They need to develop guidelines on how to work together as a team and how to include the patient and relatives into the team. They need to learn to listen to the patient and value his/her input and use their requests for assistance to shape the care they provide. They also need to coordinate both social and health care interventions together to meet the total needs of patients and relatives. (Teamwork leader 2, Canada)

A view from the UK:

There is work to be done understanding diversity, discrimination, oppression, religion, stigma, gender, ethnicity and race. We need to educate professionals so that they understand the concepts of teamwork/interprofessional working. Patients also need to know how the staff are organised and are working to use their services effectively. Furthermore, work is needed to elicit a better understanding of the key concepts of teamwork and how factors such as professional tribalism can impede it. (Teamwork leader 3, UK)

A view from the US:

I think there needs to be more grant funding and support for research and evaluation. Within both the practice and educational contexts, this should support measuring the effectiveness and maintenance of educational programmes in teaching teamwork and assessing how to use teamwork most effectively in clinical or practice settings. Another related area for research is to assess how and why some interprofessional programmes last, while others do not. What are the factors related to continuation of programmes, and how can these be 'built in' to new programmes to increase their chances of success over the long term? This type of research is more historical or longitudinal in nature. (Teamwork leader 4, US)

We need to link good theory-driven research related to teamwork with the practical quality improvement approaches. We need to test just how much of business and aviation industry concepts and experiences apply in health care; we need to make sense of all the emerging competency-based taxonomies and we also need to differentiate between different types of teamwork models intended to produce different kinds of outcomes, access to care, filling worker shortages, comprehensive care, quality and safety. (Teamwork leader 5, US)

For the five teamwork leaders, future work centres on the need to develop better local interprofessional team relations, to develop the empirical, conceptual and theoretical base for interprofessional teamwork, as well as assess the contribution that professional education systems can make to preparing professionals for teamwork.

Ways forward

Drawing upon the work presented in previous chapters we now offer a range of ways forward for interprofessional teamwork in relation to future *intervention* and *evaluation* work.

Intervening to improve interprofessional teamwork

As previously discussed, we are committed to intervening to attempt to improve teamwork, interprofessional relations and the effects of teamwork on the delivery of care. Below are a number of future directions for developing and implementing interprofessional teamwork interventions:

- There is a need for more explicit awareness and understanding of existing structural factors such as professional power and hierarchical differences in the design and development of interventions. Future intervention designs should therefore take into account how wider professional and organisational factors may influence (most likely impede) teamworking activities. Over time, more explicit attention to these factors may also trigger contextual changes such as national policies and funding arrangements which promote interprofessional teamwork. However, such change may be slow due to the conservative nature of governments and professional bodies.

- Given the scope and complexity of contextual-level interventions, these largely depend on the support of national and regional governments and professional bodies. Such interventions will depend upon a range of individuals – policy makers, practitioners, educators, researchers and consumers – who will need to work closely together over extended timeframes to develop and implement this type of large-scale intervention. In contrast, due to the focused and smaller scale nature of relational, processual and organisational interventions, these are likely to be more achievable in the short term. Individuals interested in promoting teamwork at this level should therefore focus their attention on developing *local interventions* which aim at making change at relational (e.g. team training), processual (e.g. role shifting) and organisational (e.g. reorganising care delivery) levels. Attempting to intervene at these levels is more achievable, as there is more flexibility and scope for making change and implementing efforts to improve teamwork.

- Due to the complexities of interprofessional teamwork (see Chapters 3 and 4 in particular), there is a need for future interventions to adopt a *multifaceted* approach. As we discussed in Chapter 6, combining a relational intervention such as team training with an organisational change to reconfigure ward space to support interprofessional teamwork is likely to yield more gains than the use of a single intervention.

- A key step in the design of teamwork interventions is to define the nature of the interprofessional 'problem'. The use of our *typology of interprofessional work* (see Figure 3.1) can help understand the nature of the problem, and whether it is related to teamwork, or another form of interprofessional work such as collaboration, coordination or networking. As well as helping to identify the nature of a problem, this typology can also be employed to inform the design of interprofessional interventions, which might focus on improving teamwork or coordination activities, depending upon the local context and local interprofessional needs – as outlined in our *contingency approach* and our notion of *adaptive teamwork*.

- Theory, as we discussed in Chapter 5, needs to be employed in the design and development of interprofessional teamwork interventions. The use of social science theory, in particular, can help to understand the nature of interprofessional relations, which in turn can inform activities which may be more likely to affect change. Also, the use of theory in intervention development helps its transferability from one setting to another.

Evaluating to extend our understanding of interprofessional teamwork

As well as having a shared commitment for intervening to improve interprofessional teamwork, as researchers we all share a desire to evaluate the things we do – to provide evidence for their (positive, neutral or negative) effects. Below are a number of future directions for evaluating interprofessional teamwork activities:

- There is a need for more high quality evaluations of the effects of teamwork interventions across care settings (e.g. primary, acute) and geographic locations (e.g. low- and middle-income countries). Preferably, these evaluations should adopt a *mixed methods* approach in the form of RCTs with complementary strands of qualitative and economic data.
- More thought needs to be given to generating a wider range of teamwork outcomes. Further *outcome data* are needed in the areas of staff absenteeism, staff morale, patient safety, patient care and costs-and-benefits. In addition, we need a firmer understanding of the impact of the introduction of new technologies (e.g. telemedicine, electronic patient records) on interprofessional teamwork.
- Greater exploration of interprofessional teams *in action* is needed by the use of qualitative observational approaches such as ethnography. This could include investigation of how tasks and roles are negotiated between professionals across different settings and locations, how different professionals understand what constitutes interprofessional teamwork and how informal mechanisms of interprofessional communication (such as corridor conversations) may support teamwork.
- Better evaluation of interprofessional teams is needed that includes a focus on a wider range of professions (e.g. therapists, pharmacists and social workers), as well as patients and their families.
- Further development of our *typology of interprofessional work* (see Figure 3.1) is needed to establish how our *contingency approach* and our notion of *adaptive teamwork* can and ought to be used in future. For example, if professionals only require low integration and infrequent contact in their interprofessional work, evaluation could explore how the use of a network approach might support their practice.

- There needs to be more sharing of knowledge across disciplinary areas (stroke unit teams, community mental health teams, operating room teams) to understand, with more certainty, how findings gathered from teams in one field may (or may not) translate to teams based in others.
- Lastly, but importantly, more longitudinal evaluation is needed to generate a better insight into the sustainability of teamwork interventions over time (e.g. six months, one year, five years).

References

Abbott A (1988) *The System of Professions*. University of Chicago Press, Chicago.

Accreditation Council for Graduate Medical Education (2007) *Common Program Requirements: General Competencies*. Available at: http://www.acgme.org/outcome/comp/GeneralCompetenciesStandards21307.pdf (accessed 25 July 2009).

Adair J (1986) *Effective Teamworking*. Pan, London.

Adams A, Bond S & Arber S (1995) Development and validation of scales to measure organisational features of acute hospital wards. *International Journal of Nursing Studies*; 32:612–627.

Aiken L, Buchan J, Ball J & Rafferty A-M (2008) Transformative impact of Magnet designation: England case study. *Journal of Clinical Nursing*; 17:3330–3337.

Aiken L, Smith H & Lake E (1994) Lower medicare mortality among a set of hospitals known for good nursing care. *Medical Care*; 32:771–787.

Albert M, Laberge S & Hodges BD (2009) Boundary-work in the health research field: biomedical and clinician scientist' perceptions of social science research. *Minerva*; 47:171–194.

Allen D (2002) Time and space on the hospital ward: shaping the scope of nursing practice. In D Allen & D Hughes (eds) *Nursing and the Division of Labour in Healthcare*. Palgrave, Basingstoke.

Allen N & Hecht T (2004) The 'romance of teams': toward an understanding of its psychological underpinnings and implication. *Journal of Occupational and Organisational Psychology*; 77:439–461.

American Academy of Pediatrics (2009) *National Center for Medical Home Initiatives*. Available at: http://www.medicalhomeinfo.org/index.html (accessed 15 April 2009).

Amey P, Gregson K, Johnson M, Moulster G & Nobbs M (2006) Person-centred planning: a team approach. *Learning Disability Practice*; 9:12–16.

Anderson M & Leflore J (2008) Playing it safe: simulated team training in the operating room. *AORN Journal*; 87:772–779.

Anderson N & West M (1994) *The Team Climate Inventory: Manual and Users' Guide*. ASE Press, Windsor.

Anderson N & West M (1998) Measuring climate for work group innovation: development and validation of the team climate inventory. *Journal of Organisational Behavior*; 19:235–258.

Anderson R (2008) Confidentiality and connecting for health. *British Journal of General Practice*; **58**:75–76.

Annandale E, Clark J & Allen E (1999) Interprofessional working: an ethnographic case study of emergency health care. *Journal of Interprofessional Care*; 13:139–145.

Argyris C & Schön D (1978) *Organisational Learning*. Addision-Wesley, Reading, MA.

Armstrong D (1982) The doctor-patient relationship: 1930–80. In P Wright & A Treacher (eds) *The Problem of Medical Knowledge. Examining the Social Construction of Medicine*. Edinburgh University Press, Edinburgh.

Armstrong D (1985) Space and time in British general practice. *Social Science and Medicine*; 20:659–666.

Ascano-Martin F (2008) Shift report and SBAR: strategies for clinical post conference. *Nurse Educator*; 33:190–191.

Association of American Medical Colleges (2009) *Foundations for Future Physicians*. AAMC, Washington DC.

Association of Facilities of Medicine of Canada (2007) *Accreditation of Interprofessional Health Education in Canada*. Available at: http://www.afmc.ca/projects-aiphe-e.php (accessed 6 October 2009).

Aston J, Shi E, Bullot H, Galway R & Crisp J (2005) Qualitative evaluation of regular morning meetings aimed at improving interdisciplinary communication and patient outcomes. *International Journal of Nursing Practice*; 11:206–213.

Atwal A & Caldwell K (2002) Do multidisciplinary integrated care pathways improve interprofessional collaboration? *Scandinavian Journal of Caring Science*; 16:360–367.

Audit Commission (1992) *Homeward Bound: A New Course for Community Health*. HSMO, London.

Australian Government (2008) *Towards a National Primary Health Care Strategy: A Discussion Paper from the Australian Government*. Australian Government, Canberra.

Australian Government (2009) *A Healthier Future for all Australians – Final Report of the National Health and Hospital Reform Commission*. Australian Government, Canberra.

Australian Institute of Health and Welfare (2008) *Rural, Regional and Remote Health: Indicators of Health System Performance*. Available at: http://www.aihw.gov.au/publications/phe/rrrh-ihsp/rrrh-ihsp.pdf (accessed 29 May 2009).

Awad S, Fagan S, Bellows C, Albo D, Green-Rashad B, De La Garza M & Berger D (2005) Bridging the communication gap in the operating room with medical team training. *The American Journal of Surgery*; 190:770–774.

Baker D, Gustafson F, Beaubien J, Salas E & Barach P (2005) *Medical Teamwork and Patient Safety: The Evidence-based Relation*. Agency for Healthcare Research and Quality, Rockville, MD.

Baldwin D (2007) An interprofessional celebration. *Journal of Interprofessional Care*; 21 (Suppl. 1):1–113.

Baldwin D & Daugherty S (2008) Interprofessional conflict and medical errors: results of a national multi-specialty survey of hospital residents in the US. *Journal of Interprofessional Care*; 22:573–586.

Bales R (1976) *Interaction Process Analysis: A Method for the Study of Small Groups*. University of Chicago Press, Chicago.

Bales R & Cohen S (1979) *SYMLOG: A System for Multiple Level Observation of Groups*. Free Press, New York.

Bali R (2005) *Clinical Knowledge Management: Opportunities and Challenges*. Idea Group, Hershey, PA.

Balint M (1955) The doctor, his patient and the illness. *Lancet*; 318:1.

Balint M (1956) *The Doctor, His Patient and the Illness*. Pitman, London.

Barnett-Page E & Thomas J (2009) Methods for the synthesis of qualitative research: a critical review. *BMC Medical Research Methodology*; 9:59. Available at: http://www.biomedcentral.com/1471–2288/9/59 (accessed 20 February 2010).

Barr H (1998) Competent to collaborate: towards a competency-based model for interprofessional education. *Journal of Interprofessional Care*; 12:181–188.

Barr H, Koppel I, Reeves S, Hammick M, Freeth D (2005) *Effective Interprofessional Education: Assumption, Argument and Evidence*. Blackwell, London.

Barry R, Murcko A & Brubaker C (2002) *The Six Sigma Book for Healthcare: Improving Outcomes by Reducing Errors*. Health Administration Press, Chicago.

Bass B (1997) *Transformational Leadership*. Lawrence Earlbaum Associates, Boston.

Baxter P & Markle-Reid M (2009) An interprofessional team approach to fall prevention for older home care clients 'at risk' of falling: health care providers share their experiences. *International Journal of Integrated Care*; 9:15. Available at: http://www.pubmedcentral. nih.gov/articlerender.fcgi?artid=2691945.

Beach M, Saha S & Cooper L (2006) *The Role and Relationship of Cultural Competence and Patient-centeredness in Health Care Quality*. Available at: http://www.commonwealthfund .org/usr_doc/Beach_rolerelationshipcultcomppatient-cent_960.pdf (accessed 6 October 2009).

Becker H, Geer B, Hughes E & Strauss A (1961) *Boys in White: Student Culture in Medical School*. University of Chicago Press, Chicago.

Beckman H, Markakis K, Suchman A & Frankel R (1994) The doctor-patient relationship and malpractice. Lessons from plaintiff depositions. *Archives of Internal Medicine*; 154:1365–1370.

Berwick D (2002) A user's manual for the IOM's 'Quality Chasm' report. *Health Affairs*; 21:80–90.

Biggs J (1993) From theory to practice: a cognitive systems approach. *Higher Education Research and Development*; 12: 73–85.

Bion W (1961) *Experiences in Groups and Other Papers*. Tavistock Publications, London.

Blane D (1991) Health professions. In G Scambler (ed.) *Sociology as Applied to Medicine*. Bailliere Tindall, London.

Bloor G & Dawson P (1994) Understanding professional culture in organizational context. *Organization Studies*; 15:275–295.

Blue I & Fitzgerald B (2002) Interprofessional relations: case studies of working relationships between registered nurses and general practitioners in rural Australia. *Journal of Clinical Nursing*; 11:314–321.

Blumenthal D & Kilo C (1998) A report card on continuous quality improvement. *The Milbank Quarterly*; 76:625–648.

Bodenheimer T (2005) High and rising health care costs: technologic innovation. *Annals of Internal Medicine*; 142:932–937.

Booth J & Hewison (2002) Role overlap between occupational therapy and physiotherapy during in-patient stroke rehabilitation: an exploratory study. *Journal of Interprofessional Care*; 16:31–41.

Borrill C, Carletta J, Carter A, Dawson J, Garrod S, Rees A, Richards A, Shapiro D & West M (2001) *The Effectiveness of Health Care Teams in the National Health Service*. Aston University, Birmingham.

Bourdieu P (1986) The forms of capital. In J Richardson (ed.) *Handbook of Theory and Research for the Sociology of Education*. Greenwood, New York.

Boyce R, Moran M, Nissen L, Chenery H & Brooks P (2009) Interprofessional education in health sciences: the University of Queensland Health Care Team Challenge. *Medical Journal of Australia*; 190:433–436.

Boyes A (1995) Health care assistants: delegation of tasks. *Emergency Nurse*; 3:6–9.

Brazilian Government Ministry of Health (2004) *Family Health Strategy and Primary Care.* Available at: http://dtr2004.saude.gov.br/dab/docs/publicacoes/geral/family_health_strategy.pdf (accessed 6 October 2009).

Brewer J (2000) *Ethnography: Understanding Social Research.* Oxford University Press, Oxford.

Bridges J, Meyer J, Glynn M, Bentley J & Reeves S (2003) Interprofessional care co-ordinators: the benefits and tensions associated with a new role in UK acute health care. *International Journal of Nursing Studies*; 40:599–607.

Britten N, Campbell R, Pope C, Donovan J, Morgan M & Pill R (2002) Using meta-ethnography to synthesise qualitative research: a worked example. *Journal of Health Services Research and Policy*; 7:209–215.

Broadhead R (1983) *The Private Lives and Professional Identity of Medical Students.* Transaction, Brunswick, NJ.

Bronstein L (2002) Index of interdisciplinary collaboration. *Social Work Research*; 26:113–123.

Brooker D (2005) Dementia care mapping: a review of the research literature. *The Gerontologist*; 45:11–18.

Brown R, Condor S, Mathews A, Wade G & Williams J (1986) Explaining intergroup differentiation in an industrial organization. *Journal of Occupational Psychology*; 59:273–286.

Brown S (1999) Patient-centred communication. *Annual Review of Nursing Research*; 17:85–104.

Bruce N (1980) *Teamwork for Prevention.* John Wiley, Chichester.

Buchan J (1999) Still attractive after all these years? Magnet Hospitals in a changing health care environment. *Journal of Advanced Nursing*; 30:100–108.

Busch L (1982) History, negotiation and structure in agricultural research. *Urban Life*; 11:368–384.

Butler-Sloss E (1988) *The Report of the Inquiry into Child Abuse in Cleveland.* HMSO, London.

Cadell S, Bosma H, Johnston M, Porterfield P, Cline L, Dasilva J, Fraser J & Boston P (2007) Practicing interprofessional teamwork from the first day of class: a model for an interprofessional palliative care course. *Journal of Palliative Care*; 23:273–279.

Canadian Health Services Research Foundation (2006) *Teamwork in Health Care: Promoting Effective Teamwork in Healthcare in Canada.* Canadian Health Services Research Foundation, Ottawa.

Canadian Patient Safety Institute (2008) *The Safety Competences: Enhancing Patient Safety Across the Professions.* Canadian Patient Safety Institute, Ottawa.

Careau E, Vincent C & Noreau L (2008) Assessing interprofessional teamwork in a video-conference-based tele-rehabilitation setting. *Journal of Telemedicine & Telecare*; 14:427–434.

Carpenter J & Hewstone M (1996) Shared learning for doctors and social workers. *British Journal of Social Work*; 26:239–257.

Carroll T (1999) Multidisciplinary collaboration: a method for measurement. *Nursing Administration Quarterly*; 23:86–90.

Casto M (1994) Interprofessional work in the USA. In A Leathard (ed.) *Going Interprofessional: Working Together in Health and Welfare.* Routledge, London.

Centennial College (2009) *IDEAS Network.* Available at: http://www.ideasnetwork.ca/ (accessed 3 June 2009).

Choi B & Pak A (2007) Multidisciplinarity, interdisciplinarity, and transdisciplinarity in health research, services, education and policy: promotors, barriers, and strategies of enhancement. *Clinical & Investigative Medicine*; 30:224–232.

Chopra M, Munro S, Lavis J, Vist G & Bennett S (2008) Effects of policy options for human resources for health: an analysis of systematic reviews. *Lancet*; 371:668–674.

Clark P (1997) Values in health care professional socialization: implications for geriatric education in interdisciplinary teamwork. *The Gerontologist*; 37:441–451.

Clegg S (1989) *Frameworks of Power*. Sage, London.

Cohen S & Bailey D (1997) What makes teams work: group effectiveness research from the shop floor to the executive suite. *Journal of Management*; 23:239–290.

Coiera E & Toombs V (1998) Communication behavioural in a hospital setting: an observational study. *BMJ*; 316:673–676.

College of Occupational Therapists (2000) *Code of Ethics and Professional Conduct for Occupational Therapists*. COT, London.

Cooper S, O'Carroll J, Jenkin A & Badger B (2007a) Collaborative practices in unscheduled emergency care: role and impact of the emergency care practitioner – qualitative and summative findings. *Emergency Medicine Journal*; 24:625–629.

Cooper S, O'Carroll J, Jenkin A & Badger B (2007b) Collaborative practices in unscheduled emergency care: role and impact of the emergency care practitioner – quantitative findings. *Emergency Medicine Journal*; 24:630–633.

Conn C, Jenkins P & Touray S (1996) Strengthening health management: experience of district teams in The Gambia. *Health Policy Plan*; 11:64–71.

Connolly P (1995) Transdisciplinary collaboration of academia and practice in the area of serious mental illness. *Australian and New Zealand Journal of Mental Health Nursing*; 4:168–180.

Cook M (2003) Interprofessional post-qualifying education: team leadership. In S Glen & T Leiba (eds) *Interprofessional Post-qualifying Education for Nurses*. Palgrave, Basingstoke.

Corrigan M, Cupples M, Smith S, Byrne M, Leathem C, Clerkin P & Murphy A (2006) The contribution of qualitative research in designing a complex intervention for secondary prevention of coronary heart disease in two different healthcare systems. *BMC Health Services Research*; 6:90. Available at: http://www.biomedcentral.com/1472–6963/6/90 (accessed 6 October 2009).

Cott C (1998) Structure and meaning in multidisciplinary teamwork. *Sociology of Health and Illness*; 20:848–873.

Cott C, Falter L, Gignac M & Badley E (2008) Helping networks in community home care for the elderly: types of team. *Canadian Journal of Nursing Research*; 40:19–37.

Crotty M (1998) *The Foundations of Social Research*. Sage, London.

Curley C, McEachern J & Speroff T (1998) A firm trial of interdisciplinary rounds on the inpatient medical wards. *Medical Care*; 36:S4–S12.

Davies C (1995) *Gender and the Professional Predicament in Nursing*. Open University Press, Milton Keynes.

Davis P, Lay-Yee R, Scott A, Briant R & Schug S (2003) Acknowledgement of 'no fault' medical injury: review of patients' hospital records in New Zealand. *BMJ*; 326:79–80.

Dean S (2008) *The Importance of Teamwork in Health Care Teams*. Available at: http://www.upiu.com/articles/176 (accessed 17 March 2009).

Delva D & Jamieson M (2005) *High Performance Teams in Primary Care: The Basis of Interdisciplinary Collaborative Care*. Available at: http://irc.queensu.ca/gallery/1/high-performance-teams-in-primary-care-paper.pdf (accessed 17 July 2009).

Delva D, Jamieson M & Lemieux M (2008) Team effectiveness in academic primary health care teams. *Journal of Interprofessional Care*; 22:598–611.

Department of Health (1997) *The New NHS. Modern. Dependable.* DoH, London.

Department of Health and Human Services (2003) *Rural Mental Health Outreach: Promising Practices in Rural Areas.* Department of Health and Human Services, Substance Abuse and Mental Health Services, Rockville, MD.

DiMaggio P & Powell W (1983) The iron cage revisited: institutional isomorphism and collective rationality in organizational fields. *American Sociological Review;* 48:147–160.

Di Palma C (2004) Power at work: navigating hierarchies, teamwork and webs. *Journal of Medical Humanities;* 25:291–308.

Dobson R, Henry C, Taylor J, Zello G, Lachaine J, Forbes D & Keegan D (2006) Interprofessional health care teams: attitudes and environmental factors associated with participation by community pharmacists. *Journal of Interprofessional Care;* 20:119–132.

Donabedian A (1966) Evaluating the quality of medical care. *Milbank Memorial Fund Quarterly: Health and Society;* 44:166–203.

Douglas T (1983) *Groups: Understanding People Gathered Together.* Tavistock, London.

Douglas T (2000) *Basic Groupwork.* Routledge, London.

Drinka T & Clark P (2000) *Health Care Teamwork: Interdisciplinary Practice and Teaching.* Auburn House, Westport, CT.

Durkheim E (1976) *The Elementary Forms of the Religious Life.* Allen and Unwin, London.

Dutch News (2009) Lack of teamwork bad for cancer patients. *Dutch News.* Available at: http://www.dutchnews.nl/news/archives/2009/03/lack_of_teamwork_bad_for_cance.php (accessed 11 October 2009).

Edwards C (2002) A proposal that patients be considered honorary members of the healthcare team. *Journal of Clinical Nursing;* 11:340–348.

Eichhorn S (1974) *Becoming: The Actualization of Individual Differences in Five Student Health Teams.* Monterfiore Hospital & Medical Centre, New York.

Ellingson L (2005) *Communicating in the Clinic: Negotiating Frontstage and Backstage Teamwork.* Hampton Press, Cresskill, NJ.

Elwyn G, Légaré F, Weijden T, Edwards A & May C (2008) Arduous implementation: does the Normalisation Process Model explain why it's so difficult to embed decision support technologies for patients in routine clinical practice. *Implementation Science;* 3:57. Available at: http://www.implementationscience.com/content/3/1/57 (accessed 6 October 2009).

Engeström Y, Engeström R & Vahaaho T (1999) When the center does not hold: the importance of knotworking. In S Chaklin, M Hedegaard & U Jensen (eds) *Activity Theory and Social Practice.* Aarhus University Press, Aarhus.

Espin S, Regehr G, Levinson W, Baker R & Lingard L (2006) Error or 'Act of God?': a study of patients' and operating room team members' perceptions of error definition, reporting and disclosure. *Surgery;* 139:6–14.

Eysenbach G, Powell J, Kuss O & Sa E (2002) Empirical studies assessing the quality of health information for consumers on the world wide web: a systematic review. *Journal of the American Medical Association;* 287:2691–2700.

Fairall L, Bachmann O, Zwarenstein M, Lombard C, Uebel K, van Vuuren C, Steyn D, Boulle A & Bateman E (2008) Streamlining tasks and roles to expand treatment and care for HIV: randomised controlled trial protocol. *Trials;* 9:1: Available at: http://www.trialsjournal.com/content/9/1/21.

Farrell M, Schmitt M & Heinemann G (2001) Informal roles and the stages of team development. *Journal of Interprofessional Care;* 15:281–295.

Ferlie E, Ashburner L, Fitzgerald L & Pettigrew A (1996) *The New Public Management in Action*. Oxford University Press, Oxford.

Fiorelli J (1988) Power in work groups: team members' perspectives. *Human Relations*; 41:1–12.

Firth-Cozens J (1998) Celebrating teamwork. *Quality in Health Care*; 7:S3–S7.

Firth-Cozens J (2001) Multidisciplinary teamwork: the good, bad, and everything in between. *Quality in Health Care*; 10:65–66.

Foucault M (1972) *The Archaeology of Knowledge*. Tavistock, London.

Foucault M (1978) *The History of Sexuality, Volume 1: An Introduction*. Random House, New York.

Foucault M (1979) *Discipline and Punish: The Birth of the Prison*. Penguin, Harmondsworth.

Fowler P, Hannigan B & Northway R (2000) Community nurses and social workers learning together: a report of an interprofessional education initiative in South Wales. *Health and Social Care in the Community*; 8:186–191.

Freeth D, Ayida G, Berridge E-J, Sadler C & Strachan A (2006) MOSES: multidisciplinary obstetric simulated emergency scenarios. *Journal of Interprofessional Care*; 20:552–554.

Freidson E (1970) *Profession of Medicine: A Study of the Sociology of Applied Knowledge*. Harper & Row, New York.

Friedman D & Berger D (2004) Improving team structure and communication a key to hospital efficiency. *Archives of Surgery*; 139:1194–1198.

Fuller J, Edwards J, Martinez L, Edwards B & Reid K (2004) Collaboration and local networks for rural and remote primary mental healthcare in South Australia. *Health & Social Care in the Community* 12:75–84.

Funnell P (1995) Exploring the value of interprofessional shared learning. In K Soothill, L Mackay & C Webb (eds) *Interprofessional Relations in Health Care*. Edward Arnold, London.

Gair G & Hartery T (2001) Medical dominance in multidisciplinary teamwork: a case study of discharge decision-making in a geriatric assessment unit. *Journal of Nursing Management*; 9:3–11.

Gamarnikow E (1978) Sexual division of labour: the case of nursing. In A Kuhn & A Wolpe (eds) *Feminism and Materialism*. Routledge & Kegan Paul, London.

Gardezi F, Lingard L, Espin S, Whyte S, Orser B & Baker R (2009) Silence, power and communication in the operating room. *Journal of Advanced Nursing*; 65:1390–1399.

Gazarian M, Henry R, Wales S, Micallef B, Rood E, O'Meara M & Numa, A (2001) Evaluating the effectiveness of evidence-based guidelines for the use of spacer devices in children with acute asthma. *Medical Journal of Australia*; 174:394–397.

Gelmon S, White A, Carlson L & Norman L (2000) Making organizational change to achieve improvement and interprofessional learning: perspectives from health professions educators. *Journal of Interprofessional Care*; 20:131–146.

General Medical Council (2001) *Good Medical Practice*. General Medical Council, London.

Gibbon B (1999) An investigation of interprofessional collaboration in stoke rehabilitation team conferences. *Journal of Clinical Nursing*; 8:246–252.

Ginsburg P (2004) Controlling health care costs. *New England Journal of Medicine*; 351:1591–1593.

Ginsburg L & Tregunno D (2005) New approaches to interprofessional education and collaborative practice: lessons from the organizational change literature. *Journal of Interprofessional Care*; 19:S177–S187.

Gittell J, Fairfield K, Bierbaum B, Head W, Jackson R, Kelly M, Laskin R, Lipson S, Siliski J, Thornhill T & Zuckerman J (2000) Impact of relational coordination on quality of care, postoperative pain and functioning, and length of stay: a nine-hospital study of surgical patients. *Medical Care*; 38:807–819.

Goffman E (1963) *The Presentation of Self in Everyday Life*. Penguin, London.

Goldman J, Bhattacharyya O, Zwarenstein M & Reeves S (2009) Improving the clarity of the interprofessional field: implications for research and continuing interprofessional education. *Journal of Continuing Education of the Health Professions*; 29:151–156.

Golin A & Ducanis A (1981) *The Interdisciplinary Team: A Handbook for the Education of Exceptional Children*. Aspen Systems, Rockville, MD.

Goñi S (1999) An analysis of the effectiveness of Spanish primary health care teams. *Health Policy*; 48:107–117.

Gotlib Conn L, Lingard L, Reeves S, Miller K-L, Russell A & Zwarenstein M (2009) Communication channels in general internal medicine: a description of baseline patterns for improved interprofessional collaboration. *Qualitative Health Research*; 19:943–953.

Gramsci A (1988) *A Gramsci Reader*. Lawrence and Wishart, London.

Grant S & Humphries M (2006) Critical evaluation of appreciative inquiry: bridging an apparent paradox. *Action Research*; 4:401–418.

Green J (1999) Generalisability and validity in qualitative research. *BMJ*; 391:421.

Green J & Thorogood N (2004) *Qualitative Methods for Health Research*. Sage, London.

Green L, Fryer G, Yawn B, Lanier D & Dovey S (2001) The ecology of medical care revisited. *New England Journal of Medicine*; 344:2021–2025.

Greene J & Caracelli V (1997) *Advances in Mixed-method Evaluation: The Challenges and Benefits of Integrating Diverse Paradigms. New Directions for Program Evaluation, No. 74*. Jossey-Bass, San Francisco.

Greener I (2009) Towards a history of choice in UK health policy. *Sociology of Health and Illness*; 31:309–324.

Greenwood R & Meyer R (2008) A celebration of DiMaggio and Powell (1983). *Journal of Management Inquiry*; 17:258–264.

Gregson B, Cartlidge A & Bond J (1991) *Interprofessional Collaboration in Primary Health Care Organisations*. Royal College of General Practitioners, London.

Griffiths L (1998) Humour as resistance to professional dominance in community mental health teams. *Sociology of Health and Illness*; 20:874–895.

Grimshaw J & Eccles M (2004) Is evidence-based implementation of evidence-based care possible? *Medical Journal of Australia*; 180:S50–S51.

Grimshaw J, Thomas R, Maclennan G, Fraser C, Ramsay C, Vale L, Whitty P, Eccles M, Matowe L, Shirran L, Wensing M, Dijkstra R & Donaldson C (2004) Effectiveness and efficiency of guideline dissemination and implementation strategies. *Health Technology Assessment*; 8:6. Available at: http://www.ncchta.org/execsumm/summ806.htm.

Grinspun D (2007) Healthy workplaces: the case for shared clinical decision making and increased full-time employment. *Healthcare Papers*; 7:S85–S91.

Grobler L, Marais B, Mabunda S, Marindi P, Reuter H & Volmink J (2009) Interventions for increasing the proportion of health professionals practising in rural and other underserved areas. *Cochrane Database of Systematic Reviews*; (1): CD005314.

Grol R, Bosch M, Hulscher M, Eccles M & Wensing M (2007) Planning and studying improvement in patient care: the use of theoretical perspectives. *The Milbank Quarterly*; 85:93–138.

Hacking I (2004) Between Michel Foucault and Erving Goffman: between discourse in the abstract and face-to-face interaction. *Economy and Society*; 33:277–302.

Hackman J (1983) *A Normative Model of Work Team Effectiveness. Technical Report No. 2, Research Program on Group Effectiveness*. Yale School of Organization & Management, New Haven.

Hackman J (1990) *Groups that Work (and Those That Don't): Creating Conditions for Effective Teamwork*. Jossey-Bass, San Francisco.

Hall P (2005) Interprofessional teamwork: professional cultures as barriers. *Journal of Interprofessional Care*; 19 (Suppl. 1):188–196.

Hammick M, Freeth D, Koppel I, Reeves S & Barr H (2007) A best evidence systematic review of interprofessional education. *Medical Teacher*; 29:735–751.

Handy C (1999) *Understanding Organizations*, 4th edn. Penguin, London.

Hartswood M, Procter R, Rouncefield M & Slack R (2003) Making a case in medical work: implications for the electronic medical record. *Computer Supported Cooperative Work*; 12:241–266.

Harzheim E, Duncan B, Stein A, Cunha C, Goncalves M, Trindade1 T, Oliveira M & Pinto M (2006) Quality and effectiveness of different approaches to primary care delivery in Brazil. *BMC Health Services Research*; 6:156. Available at: http://www.biomedcentral.com/1472–6963/6/156 (accessed 14 July 2009).

Haynes A, Weiser T, Berry W, Lipsitz S, Breizat A & Dellinger E (2009) A surgical safety checklist to reduce morbidity and mortality in a global population. *New England Journal of Medicine*; 360:491.

Headrick L, Wilcock P & Batalden P (1998) Interprofessional working and continuing medical education. *BMJ*; 316:771–774.

Healey A, Undre S & Vincent C (2006) Defining the technical skills of teamwork in surgery. *Quality and Safety in Health Care*; 15:231–234.

Health Canada (2003) *First Ministers' Accord on Health Care Renewal*. Health Canada, Ottawa.

Health Canada (2009) *Interprofessional Education for Collaborative Patient-Centred Practice*. Available at: http://www.hc-sc.gc.ca/hcs-sss/hhr-rhs/strateg/interprof/index-eng.php (accessed 30 June 2009).

Health Council of Canada (2009) *Teams in Action: Primary Health Care Teams for Canadians*. Health Council, Toronto.

Hean S, Macleod Clark J, Adams K, Humphris D & Lathlean J (2006) Being seen by others as we see ourselves: the congruence between the ingroup and outgroup perceptions of health and social care students. *Learning in Health & Social Care*; 5:10–22.

Heinemann G & Zeiss A (2002) *Team Performance in Health Care: Assessment and Development*. Kluwer, New York.

Helman C (2000) *Culture, Health and Illness*. Butterworth-Heinemann, Oxford.

Helmreich R, Merritt A & Wilhelm J (1999) The evolution of Crew Resource Management training in commercial aviation. *International Journal of Aviation Psychology*; 9:19–32.

Henbest R & Stewart M (1989) Patient-centredness in the consultation: a method for measurement. *Family Practice*; 6:249–253.

Henneman E, Lee J & Cohen J (1995) Collaboration: a concept analysis. *Journal of Advanced Nursing*; 21:103–109.

Henrickson S, Wadhera R, ElBardissi A, Wiegmann D & Sundt T (2009) Development and pilot evaluation of a preoperative briefing protocol for cardiovascular surgery. *Journal of the American College of Surgeons*; 208:1115–1123.

Herbert C (2005) Changing the culture: interprofessional education for collaborative patient-centered practice in Canada. *Journal of Interprofessional Care*; 19 (Suppl. 1):1–4.

Hind M, Norman I, Cooper S, Gill E, Hilton R, Judd P & Newby S (2003) Interprofessional perceptions of health care students. *Journal of Interprofessional Care*; 17:21–34.

Holman C & Jackson S (2001) A team education project: an evaluation of a collaborative education and practice development in a continuing care unit for older people. *Nurse Education Today*; 21:97–103.

Hooker R & McCaig L (2001) Use of physician assistants and nurse practitioners in primary care, 1995–1999. *Health Affairs*; 20:231–238.

Horak B, Pauig J, Keidan B & Kerns J (2004) Patient safety: a case study in team building and interdisciplinary collaboration. *Journal for Healthcare Quality*; 26 (Part 2):6–13. Available at: http://www.nahq.org/journal/ce/article.html?article_id=171.

Hugman R (1991) *Power in the Caring Professions*. Macmillan, London.

ICEBeRG – Improved Clinical Effectiveness through Behavioural Research Group (2006) Designing theoretically informed implementation interventions. *Implementation Science*; 1:4. Available at: http://www.implementationscience.com/content/1/1/4.

Ignatavicius D & Hausman K (1995) *Clinical Pathways for Collaborative Practice*. W.B. Saunders Company, Philadelphia.

Ikegami N & Campbell J (2004) Japan's health care system: containing costs and attempting reform. *Health Affairs*; 23:26–36.

Illich I (1977) *Limits to Medicine*. Penguin, New York.

Ingram H & Desombre T (1999) Teamwork in health care: lessons from the literature and from good practice around the world. *Journal of Management in Medicine*; 13 (1): 51–58.

Institute of Medicine (2004a) *Quality through Collaboration: The Future of Rural Health*. Institute of Medicine, Washington DC.

Institute of Medicine (2004b) *Keeping Patients Safe: Transforming the Work Environment of Nurses*. Washington, DC.

International Federation of Social Worker (2009) *Global Qualifying Standards for Social Work Education and Training*. Available at: http://www.ifsw.org/p38000255.html (accessed 20 February 2010).

Janis I (1982) *Groupthink: A Study of Foreign Policy Decisions and Fiascos*, 2nd edn. Houghton Mifflin, Boston, MA.

Jaques D (1998) *Learning in Groups*, 2nd edn. Kogan Page, London.

Jeffcott S & Mackenzie C (2008) Measuring team performance in healthcare: review of research and implications for patient safety. *Journal of Critical Care*; 23:188–196.

Jeffs L, Espin S, Shannon S, Levinson W & Lingard L (in review) A new way of relating: experiences associated with a team-based error disclosure simulation intervention. *Quality and Safety in Healthcare*.

Jelphs K & Dickinson H (2008) *Working in Teams*. Policy Press, Bristol.

Jewson N (1976) The disappearance of the sick-man from medical cosmology, 1770–1870. *Sociology*; 10:225–244.

Katz P (1981) Ritual in the operating room. *Ethnology*; 20:335–350.

Katzenbach J & Smith D (1993) *The Wisdom of Teams: Creating the High Performance Organization*. Harvard Business School Press, Boston.

Kelly M (2004) Qualitative evaluation research. In C Seale, G Gobo, J Gubrium & D Silverman (eds) *Qualitative Research Practice*. Sage, London.

Kenaszchuk C, Reeves S, Nicholas D & Zwarenstein M (2010) Validity and reliability of a multiple-group measurement scale for interprofessional collaboration. *BMC Health Services Research*, 10:83. Available at: http://www.biomedcentral.com/1472-6963/10/83.

Kennedy I (2001) *The Inquiry into the Management of Care of Children Receiving Complex Heart Surgery at the Bristol Royal Infirmary*. DoH, London.

Kochan T, Bezrukova K, Ely R, Jackson S, Joshi A, Jehn K, Leonard J, Levine D & Thomas D (2003) The effects of diversity on business performance: report of the diversity research network. *Human Resource Management*; 42:3–21.

Kohn L, Corrigan J & Donaldson M (2000) *To Err is Human: Building a Safer Health System*. Institute of Medicine, Washington, DC.

Koppel I (2003) *Autonomy Eroded? Changing Discourses in the Education of Health and Community Care Professionals*. Unpublished PhD Thesis, University of London.

Kramer M & Schmalenberg C (1988) Magnet hospitals: part I. Institutions of excellence. *Journal of Nursing Administration*; 18:13–24.

Kvarnström S (2008) Difficulties in collaboration: a critical incident study of interprofessional healthcare teamwork. *Journal Interprofessional Care*; 22:191–203.

Laming H (2003) *The Victoria Climbié Inquiry*. Department of Health and Home Office, London.

Larkin G (1983) *Occupational Monopoly and Modern Medicine*. Tavistock, London.

Larson C & LaFasto F (1989) *Teamwork: What Must Go Right, What Can Go Wrong*. Sage, Newbury Park, CA.

Leathard A (1994) Interprofessional developments in Britain. In A Leathard (ed.) *Going Interprofessional: Working Together for Health and Welfare*. Routledge, London.

Leathard A (2003a) Introduction. In A Leathard (ed.) *Interprofessional Collaboration: From Policy to Practice in Health and Social Care*. Brunner-Routledge, Hove.

Leathard A (2003b) Conclusion. In A Leathard (ed.) *Interprofessional Collaboration: From Policy to Practice in Health and Social Care*. Brunner-Routledge, Hove.

Lee D (2003) Interprofessional work and education: developments in Hong Kong. In A Leathard (ed.) *Interprofessional Collaboration: From Policy to Practice in Health and Social Care*. Brunner-Routledge, Hove.

Lehman A, Dixon L, Hoch J, Deforge B, Kernan E & Frank R (1999) Cost-effectiveness of assertive community treatment for homeless persons with severe mental illness. *British Journal of Psychiatry*; 174:346–352.

Lemieux-Charles L & McGuire WL (2006) What do we know about health care team effectiveness: a review of the literature. *Medical Care Research and Review*; 63:263–270.

Leonard M, Graham S & Bonacum D (2004) The human factor: the critical importance of effective teamwork and communication in providing safe care. *Quality and Safety in Health Care*; 13:85–90.

Levinson W & Lurie N (2004) When most doctors are women: what lies ahead? *Annals of Internal Medicine*; 141:471–474.

Lewin S, Glenton C & Oxman A (2009a) Use of qualitative methods alongside randomised controlled trials of complex healthcare interventions: methodological study. *BMJ*; 339:b3496.

Lewin S, Oxman A, Lavis J, Fretheim A, Marti S, Munabi-Babigumira S (2009b) SUPPORT Tools for evidence-informed health Policymaking (STP) 11: finding and using evidence about local conditions. *Health Research Policy and Systems*; 7 (Suppl. 1): S11.

Lewin S & Reeves S (in review) Enacting 'team' and 'teamwork': using Goffman's theory of impression management to illuminate interprofessional collaboration on hospital wards. *Social Science and Medicine.*

Lewin S, Skea Z, Entwistle V, Zwarenstein M & Dick J (2001) Interventions for providers to promote a patient-centred approach in clinical consultations. *Cochrane Database of Systematic Reviews*; (4): CD003267.

Lingard L, Espin S, Rubin B, Whyte S, Colmenares M, Baker G, Doran D, Grober E, Orser B, Bohnen J & Reznick R (2005) Getting teams to talk: development and pilot implementation of a checklist to promote safer operating room communication. *Quality and Safety in Health Care*; 14:340–346.

Long S (1996) Primary health care team workshop: team members' perspectives. *Journal of Advanced Nursing*; 23:935–941.

Macdonald K (1995) *The Sociology of the Professions.* Sage, London.

Mackintosh N, Berridge E-J & Freeth D (2009) Supporting structures for team situation awareness and decision making: insights from four delivery suites. *Journal of Evaluation in Clinical Practice*; 15:46–54.

Mackay L, Soothill K & Webb C (1995) Troubled times: the context for interprofessional collaboration? In K Soothill, L Mackay & C Webb (eds) *Interprofessional Relations in Health Care.* Edward Arnold, London.

MacKay S (2004) The role perception questionnaire (RPQ): a tool for assessing undergraduate students' perceptions of the role of other professions. *Journal of Interprofessional Care*; 18:289–302.

Mahmood-Yousuf K, Munday D, King N & Dale J (2008) Interprofessional relationships and communication in primary palliative care: impact of the Gold Standards Framework. *British Journal of General Practice*; 58:256–263.

Malinowski B (1948) *Magic, Science, and Religion.* Free Press, New York.

Mandy A, Milton C & Mandy P (2004) Professional stereotyping and interprofessional education. *Learning in Health & Social Care*; 3:154–170.

Mannan R, Murphy J & Jones M (2006) Is primary care ready to embrace e-health? A qualitative study of staff in a London primary care trust. *Informatics in Primary Care*; 14: 121–131.

Marris P (1986) *Loss and Change.* Routledge, London.

Marshall M, Gray A, Lockwood A & Green R (1998) Case management for people with severe mental disorders. *Cochrane Database of Systematic Reviews*; (2): CD000050.

Marshall S, Harrison J & Flanagan B (2009) The teaching of a structured tool improves the clarity and content of interprofessional clinical communication. *Quality and Safety in Health Care*; 18:137–140.

Martin V & Rogers A (2004) *Leading Interprofessional Teams in Health and Social Care.* Routledge, London.

May C, Mair F, Dowrick C & Finch T (2007) Process evaluation for complex interventions in primary care: understanding trials using the normalization process model. *BMC Family Practice*; 8:42.

McCallin A & Bamford A (2007) Interdisciplinary teamwork: is the influence of emotional intelligence fully appreciated? *Journal of Nursing Management*; 15:386–391.

McNair R, Brown R, Stone N & Sims J (2001) Rural interprofessional education: promoting teamwork in primary health care education and practice. *Australian Journal of Rural Health*; 9:S19–S26.

McPherson K, Headrick L & Moss F (2001) Working and learning together: good quality care depends on it, but how can we achieve it? *Quality in Health Care*; 10(SII):46–53.

Medical Advisory Secretariat (2008) *Ministry of Health and Long-Term Care. Aging in the Community: An Evidence-based Analysis*. Ontario Ministry of Health and Long-Term Care, Toronto.

Meerabeau L & Page S (1999) I'm sorry if I panicked you: nurses' accounts of teamwork in cardiopulmonary resuscitation. *Journal of Interprofessional Care*; 13:29–40.

Melia K (1987) *Learning and Working: The Occupational Socialisation of Nurses*. Tavistock, London.

Menzies I (1970) *The Functioning of Social Systems as a Defence Against Anxiety*. Tavistock Institute of Human Relations, London.

Merton R (1968) *Social Theory and Social Structure*. Free Press, New York.

Meuser J, Bean T, Goldman J & Reeves S (2006) Family health teams: a new Canadian interprofessional initiative. *Journal of Interprofessional Care*; 20:436–438.

Miller K-L, Reeves S, Zwarenstein M, Beales J, Kenaszchuk C & Gottlib-Conn L (2008) Nursing emotion work and interprofessional collaboration in general internal medicine wards. *Journal of Advanced Nursing*; 64:332–343.

Mohrman S, Cohen S & Mohrman A (1995) *Designing Team-based Organizations*. Jossey-Bass, San Francisco, CA.

Morey J, Simon R, Jay G, Wears R, Salisbury M, Dukes K & Berns S (2002) Error reduction and performance improvement in the emergency department through formal teamwork training: evaluation results of the MedTeams project. *Health Services Research*; 37:1553–1581.

Morgan G (1986) *Images of Organisation*. London, Sage.

Mulhall A, Kelly D & Pearce S (2004) A qualitative evaluation of an adolescent cancer unit. *European Journal of Cancer Care*; 13:16–22.

Murphy E, Dingwall R, Greatbach D, Parker S & Watson P (1998) Qualitative methods in health technology assessment: a review of the literature. *Health Technology Assessment*; 2:16. Available at: http://www.hta.ac.uk.

Nancarrow S & Mackey H (2005) The introduction and evaluation of an occupational therapy assistant practitioner. *Australian Occupational Therapy Journal*; 52:293–301.

National Bureau of Statistics of China (2009) http://www.stats.gov.cn/english (accessed 23 January 2009).

National Health Service Management Executive (1993) *Nursing in Primary Care – New World, New Opportunities*. NHSME, Leeds.

Newman J & Vidler E (2006) Discriminating customers, responsible patients, empowered users: consumerism and the modernisation of health care. *Journal of Social Policy*; 35:193–209.

Nisbet G, Hendry G, Rolls G & Field M (2008) Interprofessional learning for prequalification health care students: an outcomes-based evaluation. *Journal of Interprofessional Care*; 22:57–68.

Noblit G & Hare R (1988) *Meta-ethnography: Synthesizing Qualitative Studies*. Sage, Newbury Park, CA.

Norman I & Peck E (1999) Working together in adult community mental health services: an interprofessional dialogue. *Journal of Mental Health*; 8:217–230.

Norris S, Nichols P, Caspersen C, Glasgow R, Engelgau M, Jack L, Isham G, Snyder S, Carande-Kulis V & Garfield S (2002) The effectiveness of disease and case management for people with diabetes: a systematic review. *American Journal of Preventive Medicine*; 22:15–38.

Nursing and Midwifery Council (2002) *Code of Professional Conduct*. Nursing and Midwifery Council, London.

Oakley A (1981) Interviewing women: a contradiction in terms. In H Roberts (ed.) *Doing Feminist Research*. Routledge & Kegan Paul, London.

Oakley A, Strange V, Bonell C, Allen E & Stephenson J (2006) RIPPLE Study Team. Process evaluation in randomised controlled trials of complex interventions. *BMJ*; 332:413–416.

Obholzer A & Zagier Roberts V (eds) (1994) *The Unconscious at Work: Individual and Organisational Stress in the Human Services*. Routledge, London.

O'Cathain A, Murphy E, Nicholl J (2007) Why, and how, mixed methods research is undertaken in health services research in England: a mixed methods study. *BMC Health Services Research*; 7:85. Available at: http://www.biomedcentral.com/1472–6963/7/85.

O'Cathain A, Murphy E, Nicholl J (2008) The quality of mixed methods studies in health services research. *Journal of Health Service Research and Policy*; 13:92–98.

Office for National Statistics (2002) *General Household Survey*. UK Statistics Authority, London.

Ohlinger J, Brown M, Laudert S, Swanson S & Fofah O (2003) Development of potentially better practices for the neonatal intensive care unit as a culture of collaboration: communication, accountability, respect, and empowerment. *Paediatrics*; 111:471–481.

O'Neill O (2008) *Safe Births: Everybody's Business. An Independent Inquiry into the Safety of Maternity Services in England*. Kings Fund, London.

Ontario Nurses Association (2009) *Central Agreement 2008–2011*. Available at: http://www.ona.org/webfm_send/4932 (accessed 27 July 2009).

Onyett S (2003) *Teamworking in Mental Health*. Palgrave, Basingstoke.

Onyskiw J, Harrison M, Spady D & McConnan L (1999) Formative evaluation of a collaborative community-based child abuse prevention project. *Child Abuse & Neglect*; 23:1069–1081.

Opie A (1997) Thinking teams thinking clients: issues of discourse and representation in the work of health care teams. *Sociology of Health and Illness*; 19:259–280.

Opie A (2001) *Thinking Teams/Thinking Clients: Knowledge-based Teamwork*. Columbia University Press, New York.

Otten A (1992) The influences of the mass media on health policy. *Health Affairs*; 111–118.

Øvretveit J (1993) *Co-ordinating Community Care: Multidisciplinary Teams and Care Management*. Open University Press, Milton Keynes.

Øvretveit J (1997) Planning and managing teams. *Health and Social Care in the Community*; 5:269–276.

Oxman A, Bjørndal A, Flottorp S, Lewin S & Lindahl A (2008) *Integrated Health Care for People with Chronic Conditions*. Norwegian Knowledge Centre for the Health Services, Oslo.

Oxman A, Lavis J, Lewin S & Fretheim A (2009) SUPPORT tools for evidence-informed health policymaking (STP). 1. What is evidence-informed policymaking. *Health Research Policy and Systems*; 7 (Suppl 1):S1.

Packman W, Pennuto T, Bongar B, Orthwein J (2004) Legal issues of professional negligence in suicide cases. *Behavioral Sciences and the Law*; 22:697–713.

Paquette-Warren J, Vingilis E, Greenslade J & Newnam S (2006) What do practitioners think? A qualitative study of a shared care mental health and nutrition primary care program. *International Journal of Integrated Care*; 6:e18. Available at: http://www.ijic.org/.

Patel V, Kaufman D, Allen V, Shortlife E, Cimino J & Greenes R (1999) Toward a framework for computer mediated collaborative design in medical informatics. *Methods for Informatics in Medicine*; 38:158–176.

Patton M (1990) *Qualitative Evaluation and Research Methods*. Sage, Newbury Park, CA.

Pawson R & Tilley N (1997) *Realistic Evaluation*. Sage, London.

Peres E, Andrade A, Dal Poz M & Grande N (2006) The practice of physicians and nurses in the Brazilian Family Health Programme – evidences of change in the delivery health care model. *Human Resources for Health*; 4:25. Available at: http://www.human-resources-health.com/content/4/1/25.

Pietroni P (1994) Interprofessional teamwork: its history and development in hospitals, general practice and community care (UK). In A Leathard (ed.) *Going Interprofessional: Working Together for Health and Welfare*. Routledge, London.

Piquette D, Reeves S & Leblanc V (2009a) Interprofessional intensive care unit team interactions and medical crises: a qualitative study. *Critical Care Medicine*; 37:1251–1255.

Piquette D, Reeves S & LeBlanc V (2009b) Interprofessional ICU team interactions and medical crises: a qualitative study. *Journal of Interprofessional Care*; 23:273–285.

Pizzi L, Goldfarb N & Nash D (2001) Crew resource management and its applications in medicine. In K Shojania, B Duncan & K McDonald (eds) *Making Health Care Safer. A Critical Analysis of Patient Safety Practices. Evidence Report/Technical Assessment No 43*. Agency for Healthcare Research and Quality, Rockville.

Poissant L, Pereira J, Tamblyn R & Kawasumi Y (2005) The impact of electronic health records on time efficiency of physicians and nurses: a systematic review. *American Medical Informatics Association*; 12:505–516.

Pollard K, Miers M, Gilchrist M & Sayers A (2006) A comparison of interprofessional perceptions and working relationships among health and social care students: the results of a 3-year intervention. *Health & Social Care in the Community*; 14:541–552.

Porter S (1995) *Nursing's Relationship with Medicine*. Avebury, Aldershot.

Poulton B & West M (1993) Effective multidisciplinary teamwork in primary health care. *Journal of Advanced Nursing*; 18:918–925.

Poulton B & West M (1994) Primary health care team effectiveness: developing a constituency approach. *Health and Social Care in the Community*; 2:77–84.

Powell S (2007) SBAR: it's not just another communication tool. *Professional Case Management*; 12:195–196.

Pratt S, Mann S, Salisbury M, Greenberg P, Marcus R, Stabile B, McNamee P, Nielsen P & Sachs B (2007) Impact of CRM-based team training on obstetric outcomes and clinicians' patient safety attitudes. *Joint Commission Journal for Quality and Patient Safety*; 33:720–725.

Pritchard P (1995) Learning to work effectively in teams. In P Owens, J Carrier & J Horder (eds) *Interprofessional Issues in Community and Primary Health Care*. Macmillan, Basingstoke.

Pryor J (2008) A nursing perspective on the relationship between nursing and allied health in inpatient rehabilitation. *Disability & Rehabilitation*; 30:314–322.

Pullon S, Mckinlay E & Dew K (2009) Primary health care in New Zealand: the impact of organisational factors on teamwork. *British Journal of General Practice*; 59:191–197.

Quality Assurance Agency for Higher Education (2009) *The Quality Assurance Agency for Higher Education (QAA)*. Available at: http://www.qaa.ac.uk/default.asp (accessed 13 March 2009).

Radnor Z, Walley P, Stephens A & Bucci G (2006) *Evaluation of the Lean Approach to Business Management and Its Use in the Public Sector*. Scottish Executive Social Research, Edinburgh.

Rafferty A, Ball J & Aiken H (2001) Are teamwork and professional autonomy compatible, and do they result in improved hospital care? *Quality in Health Care*; 10 (Suppl.):S32–S37.

Rallis R & Rossman G (2003) Mixed methods in evaluation contexts: a pragmatic framework. In A Tashakkori & C Teddlie (eds) *Handbook of Mixed Methods in Social and Behavioural Research*. Sage, London.

Reeves S (2008) *Developing and Delivering Practice-Based Interprofessional Education*. VDM Publications, Munich.

Reeves S, Fox A & Hodges BD (2009a) The competency movement in the health professions: ensuring consistent standards or reproducing conventional domains of practice? *Advances in Health Sciences Education*; 14:451–453.

Reeves S & Freeth D (2003) New forms of information technology, new forms of collaboration? In A Leathard (ed.) *Interprofessional Collaboration: From Policy to Practice in Health and Social Care*. Routledge, London.

Reeves S, Freeth D, Leiba T, Glen S & Herzberg J (2006) Delivering practice-based interprofessional education to community mental health teams: understanding some key lessons. *Nurse Education in Practice*; 6:246–253.

Reeves S, Goldman J & Zwarenstein M (2009b) An emerging framework for understanding the nature of interprofessional interventions. *Journal of Interprofessional Care*; 23:539–542.

Reeves S & Lewin S (2004) Hospital-based interprofessional collaboration: strategies and meanings. *Journal of Health Services Research and Policy*; 9:218–225.

Reeves S & Lewin S with Meyer J, Glynn M (2003) *The Introduction of a Ward-based Medical Team System*. City University Research Report, London.

Reeves S & Pryce A (1998) Emerging themes: an exploratory research project of a multidisciplinary education module for medical, dental and nursing students. *Nurse Education Today*; 18:534–541.

Reeves S, Rice K, Gotlib Conn L, Miller K-L, Kenaszchuk C & Zwarenstein M (2009c) Interprofessional interaction, negotiation and non-negotiation on general internal medicine wards. *Journal of Interprofessional Care*; 23:633–645.

Reeves S, Zwarenstein M, Goldman J, Barr H, Freeth D, Hammick M & Koppel I (2008) Interprofessional education: effects on professional practice and health care outcomes. *Cochrane Database of Systematic Reviews*; (1): CD002213.

Regan de Bere S (2003) Evaluating the implications of complex interprofessional education for improvement in collaborative practice: a multidimensional model. *British Educational Research Journal*; 29:105–124.

Registered Nurses' Association of Ontario (2006) *Collaborative Practice Among Nursing Teams*. Registered Nurses' Association of Ontario, Toronto.

Rice T (1992) Containing health care costs in the United States. *Medical Care Review*; 49:19–65.

Rice Simpson K, James D & Knox G (2006) Nurse-physician communication during labor and birth: implications for patient safety. *Journal of Obstetric, Gynecologic & Neonatal Nursing*; 35:547–556.

Risser D, Rice M, Salisbury M, Simon R, Jay G & Berns S (1999) The potential for improved teamwork to reduce medical errors in the emergency department. The MedTeams Research Consortium. *Annals of Emergency Medicine*; 34:373–383.

Romanow R (2002) *Building on Values: The Future of Healthcare in Canada – Final Report*. Commission on the Future of Health Care in Canada, Saskatoon.

Royal College of Physicians and Surgeons of Canada (2005) *The CanMEDS Physician Competency Framework*. RCPSC, Ottawa.

Russell G (1990) Hospice programs and the hospice movement an investigation based on general systems theory. *The Hospice Journal*; 5:23–49.

Salaman G (2002) Understanding advice: towards a sociology of management consultancy. In T Clark & R Fincham (eds) *Critical Consulting: New Perspectives on the Management Advice Industry*. Blackwell, Oxford.

Salas E, Burke C, Bowers C & Wilson K (2001) Team training in the skies: does Crew Resource Management (CRM) training work? *Human Factors*; 43:641–674.

Salas E, Diaz Granados D, Klein C, Burke C, Stagl K, Goodwin G & Halpin S (2008) Does team training improve team performance? A meta-analysis. *Human Factors*; 50:903–933.

Salas E, Wilson K, Burke C & Wightman D (2006) Does Crew Resource Management training work? An update, an extension, and some critical needs. *Human Factors*; 48: 392–412.

Sanders T & Harrison S (2008) Professional legitimacy claims in the multidisciplinary workplace: the case of heart failure care. *Sociology of Health & Illness*; 30:289–308.

Scholes J & Vaughan B (2002) Cross-boundary working: implications for the multiprofessional team. *Journal of Clinical Nursing*; 11:399–408.

Scott J, Rundall T, Vogt T & Hsu J (2005) Kaiser Permanente's experience of implementing an electronic medical record: a qualitative study. *BMJ*; 331:1313–1316.

Schmidt I, Claesson C, Westerholm B, Nilsson L & Svarstad B (1998) The impact of regular multidisciplinary team interventions on psychotropic prescribing in Swedish nursing homes. *Journal of the American Geriatrics Society*; 46:77–82.

Schmitt, M (2001) Collaboration improves the quality of care: methodological challenges and evidence from US health care research. *Journal of Interprofessional Care*; 15:47–66.

Seale C (2003) *Media and Health*. Sage, London.

Seale C (ed.) (2004) *Health and the Media*. Blackwell, Oxford.

Sexton J, Thomas E & Helmreich L (2000) Error, stress and teamwork in medicine and aviation: cross sectional surveys. *BMJ*; 320:745–749.

Shaw M (1970) *Communication Processes*. Penguin, London.

Sherman J (2006) Achieving REAL results with six sigma. *Healthcare Executive*; 21:8–14.

Sinclair A (1992) The tyranny of a team ideology. *Organisation Studies*; 13:611–626.

Sinclair C (2000) *The Report of the Manitoba Paediatric Inquest: An Inquiry into Twelve Deaths at the Winnipeg Health Sciences Centre in 1994*. Province of Manitoba, Winnipeg.

Sinclair S (1997) *Making Doctors: An Institutional Apprenticeship*. Berg, Oxford.

Skjørshammer M (2001) Co-operation and conflict in a hospital: interprofessional differences in perception and management of conflicts. *Journal of Interprofessional Care*; 15:7–18.

Sorbero M, Farley D, Mattke S & Lovejoy S (2008) *Outcome Measures for Effective Teamwork in Inpatient Care: Final Report*. RAND Corporation, Santa Monica, CA.

South African Department of Health (2001) *The District Health System in South Africa: Progress Made and Next Steps*. Available at: http://www.capegateway.gov.za/Text/2003/district_health_system_sa.pdf (accessed 22 June 2009).

Spilsbury K & Meyer J (2004) Use, misuse and non-use of health care assistants: understanding the work of health care assistants in a hospital setting. *Journal of Nursing Management*; 12:411–418.

Stark S, Stronach I & Warne T (2002) Teamwork in mental health: rhetoric and reality. *Journal of Psychiatric and Mental Health Nursing*; 9:411–418.

Stewart M (1995) Effective physician–patient communication and health outcomes: a review. *CMAJ*; 152:1423–1433.

Stock R (2004) Drivers of team performance: what do we know and what have we still to learn? *Schmalenbach Business Review*; 56:274–306.

Strange F (1996) Handover: an ethnographic study of ritual in nursing practice. *Intensive and Critical Care Nursing*; 12:106–112.

Stroke Unit Trialists' Collaboration (2007) Organised inpatient (stroke unit) care for stroke. *Cochrane Database of Systematic Reviews*; (4): CD000197.

Strauss A (1978) *Negotiations: Varieties, Contexts, Processes and Social Order*. Jossey-Bass, San Francisco.

Strauss A, Schatzman D, Ehrlich R, Bucher M & Sabshin C (1963) The hospital and its negotiated order. In E Freidson (ed.) *The Hospital in Modern Society*. The Free Press, New York.

Strong K, Mathers C, Leeder S & Beaglehole R (2005) Preventing chronic diseases: how many lives can we save? *Lancet*; 366:1578–1582.

Stufflebeam D (2000) The CIPP model of evalution. In D Stufflebeam, G Madaus & T Kellaghan (eds) *Evaluation Models: Viewpoints on Educational and Human Service Evaluation*. Kluwer, Boston.

Sundstrom E, de Meuse K & Futrell D (1990) Work teams: applications and effectiveness. *American Psychologist*; 45:120–133.

Svensson R (1996) The interplay between doctors and nurses – a negotiated order perspective. *Sociology of Health and Illness*; 18:379–398.

Szasz G (1969) Interprofessional education in the health sciences. *Millbank Memorial Fund Quarterly*; 47:449–475.

Tajfel H & Turner J (1986) The social identity theory of inter-group behavior. In S Worchel & L Austin (eds) *Psychology of Intergroup Relations*. Nelson-Hall, Chicago.

Tashakkori A & Teddlie C (eds) (2003) *Handbook of Mixed Methods in Social and Behavioural Research*. Sage, Newbury Park, CA.

Taylor J, Blue I & Misan G (2001) Approach to sustainable primary health care service delivery for rural and remote South Australia. *Australian Journal of Rural Health*; 9: 304–310.

Tergan S, Keller T & Burkhard R (2006) Integrating knowledge and information: digital concept maps as a bridging technology. *Information Visualization*; 5:167–174.

Terkin L (2008) Arrogant, abusive and disruptive – and a doctor. *New York Times*. Available at: http://www.nytimes.com/2008/12/02/health/02rage.html (accessed 10 October 2009).

Theberge N (2008) The integration of chiropractors into healthcare teams: a case study from sport medicine. *Sociology of Health & Illness*; 30:19–34.

Thorpe K, Zwarenstein M, Oxman A, Treweek S, Furberg C, Altman D, Tunis S, Bergel E, Harvey I, Magid D & Chalkidou K (2009) A pragmatic-explanatory continuum indicator summary (PRECIS): a tools to help trial designers. *Journal of Clinical Epidemiology*; 62:464–475.

Treadwell M, Franck L & Vichinsky E (2002) Using quality improvement strategies to enhance pediatric pain assessment. *International Journal for Quality in Health Care*; 14:39–47.

Turner V (1969) *The Ritual Process: Structure and Anti-structure*. Aldine, Chicago.

Vanclay L (1996) *Training to Sustain Collaboration between General Practitioners and Social Workers*. CAIPE, London.

Van Der Walt H & Swartz L (2002) Task orientated nursing in a tuberculosis control programme in South Africa: where does it come from and what keeps it going? *Social Science and Medicine*; 54:1001–1009.

Van Maanen J & Kunda G (1989) Real feelings: emotional expression and organizational culture. *Research in Organizational Behaviour*; 11:43–103.

Varpio L, Hall P, Lingard L & Schryer C (2008) Interprofessional communication and medical error: a reframing of research questions and approaches. *Academic Medicine*; 83:S76–S81.

Velji K, Baker G, Fancott C, Andreoli A, Boaro N, Tardif G, Aimone E & Sinclair L (2008) Effectiveness of an adapted SBAR communication tool for a rehabilitation setting. *Healthcare Quarterly*; 11:72–79.

Verma S, Paterson M & Medves J (2006) Core competencies for health care professionals: what medicine, nursing, occupational therapy and physical therapy share. *Journal of Allied Health*; 35:109–115.

Vest J & Gamm L (2009) A critical review of the research literature on Six Sigma, Lean and StuderGroup's Hardwiring Excellence in the United States. *Implementation Science*; 4:35. Available at: http://www.implementationscience.com/content/4/1/35 (accessed 30 August 2009).

Vogwill V (2008) *Supporting Communication between Nurses and Physicians*. Unpublished PhD Thesis, University of Toronto.

Vygotsky L (1978) *Mind in Society: The Development of Higher Psychological Processes*. Harvard University Press, Cambridge, MA.

UK Expert Patients Programme (2009) *Expert Patients Programme Community Interest Company*. Available at: http://www.expertpatients.co.uk/public/default.aspx (accessed 30 June 2009).

Wachter R (2004) The end of the beginning: patient safety five years after 'To Err Is Human'. *Health Affairs*; W4 (Web Suppl.):534–545.

Walby S, Greenwell J, Mackay L & Soothill K (1994) *Medicine and Nursing: Professions in a Changing Health Service*. Sage, London.

Way D, Jones L & Baskerville N (2001) *Improving the Effectiveness of Primary Health Care Delivery through Nurse Practitioner/Family Physician Structured Collaborative Practice*. University of Ottawa, Ottawa.

Weingart S, Simchowitz B, Kahlert Eng T, Morway L, Spencer J, Zhu J, Cleary C, Korman-Parra J & Horvath K (2009) The You CAN campaign: teamwork training for patients and families in ambulatory oncology. *Joint Commission Journal for Quality and Patient Safety*; 35:63–71.

Wertheimer J, Roebuck-Spencer T, Constantinidou F, Turkstra L, Pavol M & Diane P (2008) Collaboration between neuropsychologists and speech-language pathologists in rehabilitation settings. *The Journal of Head Trauma Rehabilitation*; 23:273–285.

West M (1994) *Effective Teamwork*. British Psychology Society Books, Leicester.

West M (1996) *Handbook of Work Group Psychology*. Wiley, Chichester.

West M & Markiowicz L (2004) *Building Team-based Working: A Practical Guide to Organisational Transformation*. British Psychology Society/Blackwell, London.

West M & Slater J (1996) *Teamworking in Primary Health Care: A Review of its Effectiveness*. Health Education Authority, London.

Wickes D (1998) *Nurses and Doctors at Work: Rethinking Professional Boundaries*. Open University Press, Milton Keynes.

Wilcock P, Campion-Smith C & Head M (2002) The Dorset Seedcorn Project: interprofessional learning and continuous quality improvement in primary care. *British Journal of General Practice*; 52:S39–S44.

Wild D, Nawaz H, Chan W & Katz D (2004) Effects of interdisciplinary rounds on length of stay in a telemetry unit. *Journal of Public Health Management and Practice*; 10:63–69.

Williams G & Laungani P (1999) Analysis of teamwork in an NHS community trust: an empirical study. *Journal of Interprofessional Care*; 13:19–28.

Willis E (1989) *Medical Dominance: The Division of Labour in Australian Health Care*. Allen & Unwin, Sydney.

Wisborg T, Rønning T, Beck V & Brattebø G (2008) Preparing teams for low-frequency emergencies in Norwegian hospitals. *Acta Anaesthesiologica Scandinavica*; 47:1248–1250.

Witz A (1992) *Professions and Patriarchy*. Routledge, London.

Wofford M, Wofford J, Bothra J, Kendrick S, Smith A & Lichstein P (2004) Patient complaints about physician behaviors: a qualitative study. *Academic Medicine*; 79:134–138.

World Health Organization (1988) *Learning Together to Work Together*. WHO, Geneva.

World Health Organization (2005) *Preparing a Healthcare Workforce for the 21st Century. The Challenge of Chronic Conditions*. WHO, Geneva.

Wright S (1994) 'Culture' in anthropology and organizational studies. In S Wright (ed.) *Anthropology of Organizations*. Routledge, London.

Wright Mills C (1959) *The Sociological Imagination*. Oxford University Press, London.

Xyrichis A & Lowton K (2008) What fosters or prevents interprofessional teamworking in primary and community care? A literature review. *International Journal of Nursing Studies*; 45:140–153.

Yealy D, Auble T, Stone R, Lave J, Meehan T, Graff L, Fine J, Obrosky D, Edick S & Hough L (2004) The emergency department community-acquired pneumonia trial. Methodology of a quality improvement intervention. *Annals of Emergency Medicine*; 43:770–782.

Zagier Roberts V (1994) Conflict and collaboration: managing intergroup relations. In A Obholzer & V Zagier Roberts (eds) *The Unconscious at Work: Individual and Organisational Stress in the Human Services*. Routledge, London.

Ziguras S & Stuart G (2000) A meta-analysis of the effectiveness of mental health case management over 20 years. *Psychiatric Services*; 51:1410–1421.

Zuger A (2004) Dissatisfaction with medical practice. *New England Journal of Medicine*; 350:69–75.

Zwarenstein M, Bryant W & Reeves S (2003) In-service interprofessional education improves inpatient care and patient satisfaction. *Journal of Interprofessional Care*; 17:427–428.

Zwarenstein M, Goldman J & Reeves S (2009) Interprofessional collaboration: effects of practice-based interventions on professional practice and healthcare outcomes. *Cochrane Database of Systematic Reviews*; (3): CD000072.

Zwarenstein M & Reeves S (2002) Working together but apart: barriers and routes to nurse-physician collaboration. *The Joint Commission Journal on Quality Improvement*; 28:242–247.

Zwarenstein M & Reeves S (2006) Knowledge translation and interprofessional collaboration: where the rubber of evidence based care hits the road of teamwork. *Journal of Continuing Education in the Health Professions*; 26:46–54.

Zwarenstein M, Reeves S, Russell R, Kenaszchuk C, Gotlib Conn L, Miller K-L, Lingard L & Thorpe K (2007) Structuring communication relationships for interprofessional teamwork (SCRIPT): a cluster randomized controlled trial. *Trials*; 8:1. Available at: www.trialsjournal.com/content/8/1/23.

Appendices

This section of the book sets out a range of interprofessional teamwork resources aimed at providing support for readers involved in the design, implementation and evaluation of their interprofessional teamwork activities.

We offer five separate appendices:

Appendix 1 presents information on how to plan and implement an interprofessional teamwork intervention.

Appendix 2 provides methodological, practical and ethical information on how to plan and undertake an evaluation of a teamwork intervention.

Appendix 3 offers a reading list of papers and texts for those interested in critically assessing interprofessional teamwork studies.

Appendix 4 outlines a number of tools which might be employed to help evaluate teamwork activities.

Appendix 5 provides a range of online resources which offer additional information on interprofessional teamwork.

Appendix 1: Designing teamwork interventions

This appendix is divided into two main sections. The first presents information on the tools and approaches that can be employed in the planning of a teamwork intervention. The second provides a range of ideas for intervention activities that might be used to promote interprofessional teamwork.

Part 1: Intervention planning tools

We suggest three intervention tools which, although developed in other fields, resonate for the planning of interprofessional teamwork interventions.

Medical Research Council

The UK Medical Research Council provides useful guidance on the design and evaluation of complex interventions. We have summarised some questions which assist this process.

1. Intervention development:
   - Is there clarity on the intervention aims and outcomes?
   - Does the intervention have a coherent theoretical basis, which has been used systematically in the intervention development?
   - Can the intervention be described fully, so that it can be properly implemented for the purposes of evaluation and replicated by others?
   - Does the existing evidence, ideally collated in systematic review, suggest that the intervention is likely to be effective?
   - Can the intervention be implemented, and is it likely to be widely implementable if the results are favourable?

   If there is uncertainty about any of the answers posed in the questions above, further development work is needed before further progression is made.

2. Piloting and feasibility:
   - Has there been enough piloting and feasibility work to inspire confidence about the intended delivery of the intervention?

- Are there safe assumptions about intervention variability, and rates of re-cruitment and retention?

3. Evaluating the intervention:
    - Which evaluation design (see below) is going to be employed and why?
    - Are there procedures for monitoring the delivery of the intervention and overseeing the conduct of the evaluation?

A qualitative (process) evaluation is recommended by the Medical Research Council (MRC) to explain discrepancies between expected and observed out-comes, to understand how contextual influences may affect outcomes and to provide insights to aid further implementation. It also recommends that an economic evaluation is included in order to make evaluation findings more useful for decision-makers.

4. Reporting: The MRC recommends that a report of the intervention is pro-vided, which includes full details on methods and findings. This, it is noted, helps to enable replication studies or wider scale implementation.

5. Implementation: Strategies to encourage implementation of evaluation find-ings should be undertaken. These need to be based on a scientific under-standing of the behaviours that need to change, relevant decision-making processes, and the barriers and facilitators of change. If the intervention is translated into routine practice, monitoring should be undertaken to detect adverse events or long-term outcomes that could not be observed directly in the original evaluation; or to assess whether the effects observed in the study are replicated in routine practice.

For more information on this tool see: Medical Research Council (2008) *Devel-oping and Evaluating Complex Interventions: New Guidance*. MRC, London. Available at: http://www.mrc.ac.uk/Utilities/Documentrecord/index.htm?d=MRC004871 (accessed 21 February 2010).

SUPPORT tools

Fretheim *et al*. (2009) provide informative advice about the planning and imple-mentation of policies and programmes, which is helpful in developing and im-plementing interprofessional teamwork interventions. They state that a key issue related to the design of an intervention rests upon a comprehensive consideration of potential barriers to its successful implementation. They outline a number of issues that need to be examined, including eliciting the views of relevant stake-holder groups in order to identify potential barriers, considering the use of dif-ferent organisational strategies such as management support for the intervention, and exploring the use of changes in local policies and procedures as an inexpen-sive and potentially effective means of eliciting change.

For more information on this tool see: Fretheim A, Munabi-Babigumira S, Oxman A, Lavis J & Lewin S (2009) SUPPORT Tools for evidence-informed policymaking in health 6: using research evidence to address how an option will be implemented. *Health Research Policy and Systems*; 7 (Suppl. 1):S6.

NorthStar

This is a tool that aims to support the development of interventions aimed at improving the quality of care. Its target audience includes researchers, health care professionals and managers responsible for developing, delivering and evaluating continuing education and quality-improvement interventions. It consists of a number of sections that cover the design and evaluation of interventions.

For more information on this tool see: Akl E, Treweek S, Foy R, Francis J, Oxman A (2007) NorthStar – a support tool for the design and evaluation of quality improvement interventions in healthcare. *Implementation Science*; 19:2. Available at: http://www.implementationscience.com/content/2/1/19.

Intervening with interprofessional teams

Based on the ideas in the tools presented above, as well as experiences gained from our own work, we offer below some examples of the multiple actions that are included in the development of an intervention to promote interprofessional teamwork:

- Define the problem that the teamwork intervention aims to address. This might involve identifying issues (e.g. miscommunication) which are creating deficiencies or inefficiencies in the delivery of care. This is important during the first stage, as a problem thought to be the consequence of inadequate teamworking may have a different cause or may have multiple causes.
- Define current providers of care for a group of patients, and establish both the current roles and activities of each provider and communication pathways between them.
- Negotiate with affected participants (e.g. professionals, managers, patients) to select and 'test' new approaches to one or many of the following elements: organisation of the work process; communication within a group of professionals; adding a new role to the team; redefining the team, including professionals and non-professionals; establishing new interprofessional communication processes; reallocating responsibilities and establishing accountabilities and goals.
- Select a mix of those changes or interventions that appear to promise improvements in teamworking and that are acceptable to participants, including professionals, managers, patients and others who may be affected.
- Test the innovations on a small scale and then, with modifications, on a larger scale, compared with some alternative approach or to 'usual care' approaches.

- Attempt to assess cost and effectiveness of the intervention in relation to other possible teamwork intervention options.
- Feedback key findings to key participants and decision-makers.

We next offer a synthesis of the ideas and guidance presented above to provide a checklist for interprofessional team interventions:

1. Is the intervention clearly described, including how to implement it in practice (e.g. engaging stakeholders, identifying champions)? Is it tailored to meet local conditions?
2. What focus does the intervention aims to address – relational, processual, organisational and/or contextual factors?
3. Who is/are the intervention target(s) – individual professionals, teamwork processes, organisation of care?
4. Does the intervention focus only on improving teamworking, or does it promote a range of changes of which teamworking is one?
5. How does the intervention consider the nature of power imbalances and hierarchies that operate within an interprofessional team?
6. Was the intervention developed by an interprofessional group?
7. Is the intervention informed by theory?
8. Are there explicit and measurable outcomes associated with the intervention?
9. How will the intervention be evaluated?
10. Does the intervention use formal as well as informal activities?

Part 2: Intervention activities

Next, we outline a range of activities which might be included as part of a teamwork intervention. Given that multifaceted interventions involving a range of relational, processual, organisational and contextual activities are more likely to yield results than a single activity, we encourage the use of at least two of these activities (preferably with others) when designing an intervention.

Understanding the nature of interprofessional interactions

Porter's (1995) work based on ethnographic observations of doctor–nurse interactions in an intensive care setting revealed four types of interactions used by nurses when communicating with their medical colleagues:

- Unproblematic subordination – an unquestioning approach to requests from colleagues
- Informal covert decision-making – where there is refrain from open disagreement but some informal and covert attempt at influencing clinical decision-making

- Informal overt decision-making – open informal involvement in clinical decision-making
- Formal overt decision-making – where input into clinical decision-making is encouraged to be open and colleagues discuss various options.

Through observation of team interactions, this typology could help team members to identify the nature of their interactions in a more comprehensive manner. If, for example, a team sees that there is a tendency to engage in the first type of interaction (unproblematic subordination), work could be undertaken to move them towards the fourth type (formal overt decision-making).

Developing a team policy

Øvretveit (1997) argues that teams need to spend time undertaking preparatory work to achieve clarity around team roles, responsibilities and goals. Such preparation can provide a team with opportunities to agree how to coordinate their collaborative work in an efficient and mutually satisfying manner. An important outcome of this preparation work is that teams develop a *team policy*, which explicitly records the collective aims, roles and responsibilities of the team. It also helps to ensure that a team has a formal document that provides members with details of how they operate. Øvretveit saw that each team policy should contain a number of key elements:

- An outline of the overall purpose of the team
- Information on team membership
- Clarification of individuals' roles within the team
- Details on the processes of teamwork
- Shared targets/milestones.

For Øvretveit, ongoing discussion between team members is required to ensure that their team policy is regularly updated and amended if, for example, a new member joins, and there is a need modify a previously agreed policy.

Situation–Background–Assessment–Recommendation (SBAR)

SBAR can offer a mechanism for structuring conversations, focusing on immediate attention and action. It defines four domains of content for communication between nurses and physicians, and matching physician approaches with nursing ones. SBAR helps generate a set expectations about what will be communicated between team members. This can be useful for developing team processes and fostering a culture of patient safety (Leonard *et al.*, 2004). The SBAR tool was developed by the military and the aviation industry as a method that aimed to decrease the amount of risks associated with miscommunication (Ascano-Martin, 2008). It has been described as a *'practical roadmap'* for important communication (Powell, 2007). Velji *et al.* (2008) found that SBAR has been successfully applied to health care settings such as operating rooms, intensive care units and emergency rooms, and has been shown to improve staff and patient satisfaction, team communication and clinical outcomes. More recent work has modified this tool to provide more focus content and clarity of team referrals (Marshall *et al.*, 2009).

The SBAR tool can be downloaded from the Institute for Healthcare Improvement at: http://www.ihi.org/ihi.

Team reflection activities

For West (1996), a team that can spend time together reflecting upon their collaborative work can develop a 'reflexive' (e.g. integrated and well coordinated) way of working together. As West (1996, p. 13) stated:

> Reflexivity involves the members of the team standing back and critically examining themselves, their processes and their performance to communicate about these issues and to make appropriate changes.

West identifies that the development of a reflexive team approach can help ensure that members are able to adapt and respond effectively to any changes they encounter. This is an important quality to have for health and social care teams, as change is an ongoing factor that needs to be managed by students and staff. A key aspect to achieving a reflexive approach is the creation of an environment where members value one another's contributions, feel safe to openly share their ideas and trust one another to acknowledge their shortfalls and mistakes. While West noted that the development of a reflexive approach to teamwork will take team members both time and effort, the benefit gained from this input is worthwhile. Opie (1997) stated teams who have time to reflect upon their performance are more likely to fuse together the differing knowledge bases and perspectives that each member brings to the team. A fusing process can ultimately provide a richer form of team collaboration.

Team activities aim to prevent, detect and rectify errors

O'Neill (2008) outlined a range of activities designed to prevent, detect and rectify errors which might form a series of useful interprofessional team activities:

- Identify the protocol to be used or develop a plan – it must be clear to everyone on the team what protocol or plan is being used
- Prioritise tasks for a patient – team members must understand how their individual tasks fit into the overall task
- Speak up – professionals must be prepared to speak up when patients are at risk and team leaders must foster a climate which makes this possible
- Cross-monitor within the team – team members should watch each other for errors and problems; this should be seen not as criticism but as support for fellow members and an additional defence for patients

- Give and accept feedback – feedback should not be restricted to team leaders; any member should be able and prepared to give feedback to any other. But for this to be helpful, team members need to understand each other's roles
- Use closed loop communications – communications must be acknowledged and repeated by their recipients and even their senders. This provides an additional check and defence
- Back up other team members – members need to be aware of each other's actions and be ready to step in with support and assistance.

Interprofessional negotiation

Zwarenstein & Reeves (2002) have outlined four key tasks to help ensure smooth and well-coordinated teamwork between members:

1. Agree on a shared definition of patient well-being which incorporates ideas the different perspectives of team members.
2. Identify the information to be shared in order to allow other professionals to work, and agree how this is to be shared. Define the work each profession does alone and does together.
3. Understand the differing demands and pressures each profession faces in delivering care. This can help lead to mutual support between team members.
4. Acknowledge that delivering care is difficult, not always successful and can cause anxiety.

As outlined above, this approach offers a set of practice guidelines, in the form of four simple team tasks, to encourage an interprofessional team to work in a more effective manner.

Team mind mapping

Team mind mapping is an approach which allows the graphic reconstruction of shared team knowledge. It has been argued that increasingly complex environments in education and work settings combined with high-density information requires new learning and knowledge retention strategies (Tergan *et al.*, 2006). Mind mapping is a way of helping organise information via diagrammatic branches. At the centre is the topic to be explored. Branches labelled with key words indicating major issues to be considered radiate from the centre. This activity may be used by interprofessional team members to introduce new concepts or explore important areas related to interprofessional teamwork.

Appendix 2: Evaluating interprofessional teamwork

In this appendix we provide ideas about how one can plan and implement an evaluation of interprofessional teamwork. We go on to outline a variety of key methodological, practical and ethical issues which need to be considered when designing or undertaking an interprofessional teamwork evaluation.

Methodological considerations

Below we describe and briefly discuss a number of central methodological considerations, including the use of evaluation models, selection of an evaluation design and dissemination issues.

Purpose of the evaluation

As we noted in Chapter 6, evaluations of teamwork activities can be undertaken for a variety of purposes, including assessing the effects of a new interprofessional intervention, comparing costs and benefits of one teamwork intervention with another and exploring interprofessional team processes. A clear idea of the purpose of the evaluation is crucial. Time should therefore be spent formulating a concise evaluation question, as this will provide direction for the evaluation design and the use of appropriate evaluation methods.

The use of evaluation models

While there are a variety of different models available which can help frame an evaluation, most models focus on measuring outcomes. For us, such a focus overlooks a number of other important components of an intervention, such as understanding the nature of the context in which an intervention is undertaken and also exploring the processes associated with an intervention. We therefore recommend the use of a model which adopts a comprehensive approach to evaluation such as the CIPP (Context, Input, Process, Product) evaluation model (Stufflebeam, 2000). The value of the CIPP model is that it takes into consideration the whole context

surrounding an intervention as well as the nature of the intervention and its associated outcomes.

Other similar models include Biggs's (1993) Presage-Process-Product and
Pawson & Tilley's (1997) Realistic Evaluation. Both these models have an inclusive
approach to evaluation which incorporates investigation of context, processes and
outcomes.

Evaluation designs

As noted in Chapter 6, there are a number of quantitative and qualitative evaluation designs available for use as well as the option to combine approaches to
produce a mixed methods evaluation. In this section we review each of the main
evaluation designs.

Below are the main quantitative evaluation designs which can be employed.

Randomised control trials

This type of design randomly selects participants for inclusion in either the intervention or control groups. Randomised control trials (RCTs) can provide a rigorous understanding of the nature of change associated with an intervention.
The randomisation of individuals reduces bias related to selection or recruitment.
As the effects of most complex interventions, such as those aimed at changing
teamwork practice, are modest, of the order of 10% improvements, perhaps even
smaller. The detection of such small differences is made easier if an RCT is used to
help distinguish the effects of the intervention from other potential causes.

Cluster RCTs

In situations where the intervention naturally operates at the level of a team, or
where some patients cannot be removed from the effects of an intervention, it
is often possible to randomise intact units (such as wards or practices), known
as 'clusters'. These trials are known as cluster randomised trials. Randomising in
clusters is administratively and logistically easier in these situations, reduces con-
tamination, and may, especially for teamwork interventions, be the natural level of
application of interventions. For example, wards can be selected as the experimental unit in trials evaluating interprofessional collaboration initiatives (e.g. Zwarenstein *et al.*, 2007). Such trials can seldom be undertaken within a single institution,
as there are rarely sufficient clusters to randomise.

Controlled before and after studies

This design adopts a similar approach to an RCT, but does not randomise who
receives the intervention. While this type of design can usefully measure change,
it cannot assess whether reported outcomes are sustained over time. Nevertheless,
a well-matched control should give a sense of secular trends and sudden changes,

and should be attempted if an RCT or interrupted time series (see below) is not possible.

Interrupted time series studies

This is a non-randomised design that uses multiple measurements before and after a teamwork intervention to determine if it has an effect that is greater than the underlying trend. This design usually requires multiple time points before the intervention to identify any underlying trends or any cyclical phenomena, and multiple points afterwards to see if there is any change in the trend measured previously. Interrupted time series studies do not control for outside influences on outcomes. They are also difficult to undertake in settings where routine outcome data are not collected.

Before-and-after study

This is a non-randomised design where the evaluator collects data before and after a teamwork intervention. This design helps detect changes resulting from an intervention more accurately as there is data collection at two points in time: before and after the intervention. Despite gathering data at two time points, this design is still limited in providing a rigorous understanding of change, as it cannot say accurately whether the change was attributable to the intervention or another confounding influence.

Below are the main qualitative evaluation designs which can be employed:

Ethnography

Ethnography is the study of social interactions, behaviours and perceptions that occur within teams, organisations, networks and communities. The central aim of ethnography is to provide rich, holistic insights into people's views and actions, as well as the nature of the social setting they inhabit, through the collection of detailed observations and interviews.

Grounded theory

This is an approach that is used to explore social processes that are present within human interactions. Grounded theory differs from other approaches in that its primary purpose is to develop a theory about dominant social processes rather than to describe particular phenomena. Through its application researchers are able to develop explanations of key social processes that are grounded or derived in the data.

Phenomenology

This form of inquiry focuses on individuals' perceptions of their experience with all types of phenomena. Phenomenology is both a philosophy and research approach that allows for the exploration and description of phenomena important to health and social care teams. The goal of phenomenology is to describe 'lived experience'.

Action research

Action research is known by various names, including cooperative learning, participatory action research and collaborative research. Action research is a form of inquiry which involves people in a process of change, which is based on professional, organisational or community action. It adopts a more collaborative approach than the designs described above, where evaluators play a key role with participants in processes of planning, implementing and evaluating change.

As noted above, there is also the possibility of combining quantitative and qualitative approaches:

Mixed methods

As noted in Chapter 6, mixed methods evaluation aim to gather different types of quantitative and qualitative data (e.g. surveys, interviews, documents, observations) to provide a more detailed understanding of the processes and outcomes associated in an intervention. Triangulation between quantitative and qualitative data can help generate more insightful empirical findings.

Influence of the evaluator

One needs to acknowledge the influence of the evaluator in their empirical work. In quantitative evaluation, the main influence is in the framing of the questions and identifying the contexts or populations to be studied. In qualitative evaluation, where the evaluator becomes immersed in the data, they are the main influence. Across both types of evaluation one needs to remember that the evaluator can also influence the boundaries of the study, the evaluation design, data collection methods and the approach to data analysis.

Internal and external evaluations

An 'insider' evaluator can benefit from extensive knowledge of the history and context of a study setting, but this can make it difficult for them to stand back from the data and interpret it in a detached manner. By contrast, external evaluators may find it easier to view their work from a more neutral viewpoint. This neutrality is also helpful for eliciting more candid data from participants. However, external evaluators often have to spend time developing an in-depth understanding of contextual issues. External evaluations are also often accorded greater influence because they are seen as more 'impartial'.

Reactivity

Reactivity is a term used to describe a phenomenon where the presence of the evaluator positively changes research participants' behaviour – also known as *The Hawthorne Effect*. Assessing the level of reactivity on an evaluation study is difficult, but one needs to be aware of its presence and its possible effects. Over time, reactivity issues diminish, as individuals cannot usually alter their behaviour – in the presence of an evaluator – for extended periods of time.

Dissemination issues

Disseminating findings from a study is a critical part of the evaluation process. It provides key stakeholders (participants, managers, employers, funders, patients, fellow evaluators) with important information about the effects of a certain intervention. It can also provide these stakeholders with insights into how they might achieve similar successes in their own work. There are a number of different routes of dissemination to consider. These include:

- Local meetings – useful for formative, internal evaluation work
- National or international conferences/meetings (posters, papers) – these are useful places to discuss early work to elicit feedback on processes and/or outcomes
- Short reports in professional journals – these are particularly useful for describing work in progress and/or directing readers to a more lengthy report
- Peer reviewed papers – these can provide more information on the intervention and evaluation, usually for an academic audience
- Websites – these can provide rapid, easily updated, low-cost access to evaluation information. Feedback can also be obtained from those who use the site.

Key messages from one's evaluation should be disseminated as widely as possible. Therefore, it is useful to consider undertaking local presentations as well as presentations at national or international conferences. In addition, one should attempt to publish work via professional and/or academic journals.

Practical considerations

Below we consider a number of key practical issues related to evaluating interprofessional teamwork activities, including obtaining access to study sites and managing multiple stakeholders.

Obtaining access

Obtaining access into a study site is a key step in the implementation of an evaluation. If an evaluation aims to gather data from staff or patients, there will be several gatekeepers, such as senior physicians, nurses and service managers who need to be approached to gain their approval.

Managing stakeholders

Evaluation often involves a wide range of stakeholders with an interest in the conduct and findings of the evaluation. Evaluation aims and methods may need to be negotiated with these groups. However, they may have little knowledge of research methodology and may not always reach agreement among themselves.

Prepare for change

Change is a constant factor that exists in all health and social care systems. As a result, the evaluation of interventions in the real world is difficult to contain and control, as both context and intervention may be changing as the evaluation progresses. New policies may be implemented that influence teamworking in the implementation or comparison sites, or the teamwork intervention may be stopped if managers have to contend with new priorities. In addition, evaluations are often limited by a range of local changes, such as time and funding constraints, or the loss of a local teamwork champion which can undermine ongoing evaluation work (Lewin *et al.*, 2009b).

Politics

Evaluation can be a highly political activity. For example, granting agencies may disagree on the interpretation of findings or may reject them. Evaluations can also be commissioned to support decisions that have already been taken, or interventions can be implemented with only limited evaluation evidence. For instance, mental health case management was adopted by the UK government as a policy even though limited evidence existed on its effects (e.g. Marshall *et al.*, 1998). In addition, management may not go on to implement an intervention which has generated positive findings from pilot work.

Considering the resources

Finding time and money for evaluating interprofessional teamwork can be difficult. Wherever possible, one should consider how to secure funding for all stages of the evaluation process, including literature reviewing, question formulation, selection of designs, ethical approval, data collection/analysis and dissemination of findings. Substantially more funds are needed to evaluate larger-scale, longer-term work that can chart multi-levelled change in complex environments.

Ethical considerations

Evaluation work must be undertaken on an ethical basis. As evaluations of interprofessional teamwork activities involve humans, ethical clearance is required. An attention to ethics is critical, as it ensures individuals can make an informed choice about whether (or not) they wish to participate in the evaluation, that there is no coercion related to people becoming involved, that data are anonymised (so that no one individual can be identified and potentially harmed) and that all data are stored securely to ensure confidentiality.

However, if an evaluation aims to gain information for internal quality improvement purposes and will not be disseminated to external audiences, ethical approval may not be required. If one wishes to disseminate work further, it is recommended that ethical approval is obtained from all relevant research ethics committees.

Evaluation checklist

Below we summarise the main issues we have discussed in this appendix to provide an interprofessional teamwork evaluation checklist.

Methodological issues

- What is to be evaluated and why?
- Which conceptual model will underpin the evaluation?
- Which evaluation design will be employed – quantitative, qualitative or mixed methods?
- Who will be undertaking the evaluation – internal or external evaluator?
- How will one deal with reactivity and other biases such as evaluator influence?
- What is the dissemination plan?

Practical issues

- Is there a clear plan regarding access of study sites? Who are the key gate-keepers?
- How have stakeholders been involved in the evaluation development and implementation?
- What are the costs – financial, resources and time to – undertake the evaluation; and what resources are available for the use of the evaluation?

Ethical issues

- Has there been consideration of all ethical dimensions? Is ethical approval secured?

As we illustrate above, engaging in evaluation work involves consideration of an array of different (but interconnected) methodological, practical and ethical issues. Careful thought is required with each, as for example, a methodological decision taken about the use of a certain evaluation designs will have practical and ethical implications.

Further reading

Below are two general evaluation texts which provide some useful further reading on this subject:

Gomm R, Needham G & Bullman A (eds) (2000) *Evaluating Research in Health and Social Care*. Sage, London.

Rossi P, Lipsey M & Freeman H (2004) *Evaluation: A Systematic Approach*. Sage, London.

Appendix 3: Critical appraisal

There are a number of useful materials that can be employed to critically appraise the quality of one's own (and others') teamwork evaluations. In this appendix we present qualitative, quantitative and mixed methods approaches to critical appraisal.

Qualitative appraisal

Spencer L, Ritchie J, Lewis J & Dillon L (2003) *Quality in Qualitative Evaluation: A Framework for Assessing Research Evidence*. Government Chief Social Researcher's Office, London.

Kuper A, Lingard L & Levinson W (2008) Critically appraising qualitative research. *BMJ*; 337:687–689.

Quantitative appraisal

Duffy J (2005) Critically appraising quantitative research. *Nursing and Health Sciences*; 7:281–283.

Mixed methods appraisal

Pluye P, Gagnon M, Griffiths F & Johnson-Lafleur J (2009) A scoring system for appraising mixed methods research. *International Journal of Nursing Studies*; 46:529–546.

O'Cathain A, Murphy E & Nicholl J (2008) The quality of mixed methods studies in health services research. *Journal of Health Service Research and Policy*; 13: 92–98.

Online resources

The Critical Appraisal Skills Programme (CASP) has helped to develop an evidence-based approach in health and social care, working with local, national and international partner organisations. CASP aims to put knowledge into practice by learning how to systematically formulate questions, find research evidence, appraise and act on evidence. Four 'Crib Sheets' are available for download on evaluating randomised control trials, economic evaluations, qualitative research and systematic reviews (see http://www.casp-birmingham.org/).

Appendix 4: Tools to evaluate interprofessional teamwork

Below are a number of quantitative tools that have been developed for the evaluation of interprofessional teamwork. While, as we discussed in Chapter 6, such tools have their limitations, they may be useful as part of a mixed method evaluation which combines data generated from their use with qualitative sources.

Team Climate Inventory

This tool was developed by Anderson and West (1994, 1998) as a set of four separate but interrelated scales which aim to measure different aspects of collaborative work. First, 'team objectives' – a 13-item scale focused on clarity of team objectives and members' commitment to team objectives. Second, 'team participation' – a 12-item scale focused on team members' attitudes to cohesion and participation. Third, 'quality' – a seven-item scale focused on the extent to which team members promote quality in their teamwork processes. Fourth, 'support for innovation' – an eight-item scale focused on the amount of effort and resources given for implementing innovation.

Aston Team Performance Inventory

This tool was developed to examine the factors influencing team effectiveness in three areas by assessing the main inputs or contextual factors that influence team functioning; team and leadership processes; and the team's overall performance. The Aston Team Performance Inventory (ATPI) can be administered electronically or manually. The tool, it is claimed, is suitable for a range of teams. For more information see: www.astonod.com/atpiView.php?page=1.

Team Effectiveness Questionnaire

Developed by Poulton and West (1993, 1994), this tool has 25 items and aims to measure how 'effective' a team is in relation to four dimensions: teamwork (communication strategies, collaborative working, valuing others' roles), organisational efficiency (clear procedures, innovative practice, keeping within budgets), health care practices (staff development, research-based practice, equal opportunities) and patient-centred care (provision of information, clinical competence).

Interprofessional Collaboration Scale

This 13-item scale aims to measure perceptions of interprofessional collaboration between nurses, physicians and other health professionals. The items were written from the perspective of respondent groups to name other professionals as targets of the item concepts (e.g. 'nurses have a good understanding with physicians about our respective responsibilities'). Items were adapted from the Nurses' Opinion Questionnaire (Adams *et al.* 1995). The scale's items were written in a round-robin format to specify 'target' groups and 'rater' groups. The three underlying subscales address communication with other groups, accommodation and isolation/autonomy (Kenaszchuk *et al.*, 2010).

System for Multiple Level Observation of Groups

Developed by Bales and Cohen (1979), this tool is a 26-item rating scale that aims to measure individuals' behaviours based on three dimensions: prominence (dominance and assertiveness); sociability (warmth, friendliness) and task orientation (rationality towards tasks and task-focus).

Interaction Process Analysis

The Interaction Process Analysis tool was developed by Bales (1976) to categorise and understand the nature of interaction within groups or teams. The observation of interaction is based on assigning behaviour to a number of categories including agreeing/disagreeing, giving/asking for suggestions and giving/asking for opinions. In recording interaction between group members within these categories, this tool aims to understand the issues and processes around communication, control and decision-making.

Collaborative Practice Questionnaire

Developed by Way *et al.* (2001) in a primary care context, this scale aims to assess perceptions of collaborative practice between health and social care professions. The scale has nine items focused on communication, decision-making, coordination and collaboration.

Index of Interdisciplinary Collaboration

This scale aims to measure perceptions of collaboration by the use of 42 items which are based on five subscales focused on interdependence, newly created professional activities, flexibility, collective ownership of goals, reflection on process (Bronstein, 2002).

Multidisciplinary Collaboration

Carroll (1999) developed this scale to measure perceptions of collaboration based on 18 vignettes which are rated on a five-point Likert scale. Each vignette contains four questions linked to four subscales focused on general collaboration, patient care processes, communication and teamwork.

Interprofessional Perception Scale

Developed by Golin and Ducanis (1981), this 15-item scale aims to elicit perceptions of one's own profession as well as perceptions of other health and social care professions.

Role Perception Questionnaire

Designed by MacKay (2004), this 20-item scale aims to measure different health and social care professionals' perceptions of their own and others' roles.

The Team Survey

Developed within a primary care context by Delva and Jamieson (2005), this tool has 25 items. Questions are based on the following four factors: team identification and communication, meta-cognition of team goals and performance, team potency and shared mental models of team roles.

Further reading

Also, see Heinemann and Zeiss (2002) for further information on the use of quantitative evaluation scales designed for the evaluation of teamwork.

Appendix 5: Online resources

In this appendix we provide information on organisations which promote inter-professional teamwork as well as details on other useful teamwork websites.

Organisations that promote teamwork

As we discussed in Chapter 1, we have witnessed an expansion of organisations which champion interprofessional teamwork, collaboration and education. This section outlines a number of these organisations and provides links to their websites.

American Interprofessional Health Collaborative

The American Interprofessional Health Collaborative (AIHC) offers a venue for health and social professions based in the US to share information, mentor and support one another as they provide leadership to help influence system change with the implementation of interprofessional education and practice at their individual institutions and organisations. Website: http://blog.lib.umn.edu/cipe/aihc/

Australasian Interprofessional Practice and Education Network

Australasian Interprofessional Practice and Education Network (AIPPEN) aims to provide a forum for sharing of information, networks and experiences in the area of interprofessional practice and education in health and social care contexts across Australia and New Zealand. Website: http://www.aippen.net/

Canadian Interprofessional Health Collaborative

The Canadian Interprofessional Health Collaborative (CIHC) is a Canadian organisation that provides health providers, teams and institutions with the resources and tools needed to apply an interprofessional, patient-centred and collaborative approach to healthcare. The CIHC's core activities are designed to support individuals and institutions when they require expert advice, knowledge or information on interprofessional collaboration. Website: http://www.cihc.ca/

Centre for the Advancement of Interprofessional Education

Founded in 1987, Centre for the Advancement of Interprofessional Education (CAIPE) is dedicated to the promotion and development of interprofessional education with its individual and corporate members, and in collaboration with other organisations in the UK and overseas. It provides information and advice through its website, bulletins and papers, and has a close association with the *Journal of Interprofessional Care* (see below). CAIPE also organises workshops which facilitate development in interprofessional learning and teaching, and foster exchange and mutual support between its members and others. Website: http://www.caipe.org.uk/

European Interprofessional Education Network

European Interprofessional Education Network (EIPEN) aims to establish a sustainable inclusive network of people and organisations in partner countries to share and develop effective interprofessional learning and teaching for improving collaborative practice and multi-agency working in health and social care. EIPEN has two interlinked goals: To develop a transnational network of universities and employers and to promote good practices in interprofessional education in health and social care. Website: http://www.eipen.org/

Institute for Healthcare Improvement

The Institute for Healthcare Improvement (IHI) aims to build the will for change, cultivating concepts for improvement, and helping professions and managers implement ideas into action. The IHI also works to change the skills, attitudes and knowledge of the health and social care professions through life-long learning. A key aim of which is to reduce professional isolation, improve collaboration and the well-being of patients and their families. Website: http:// www.ihi.org/IHI/

Nordic Interprofessional Network

Nordic Interprofessional Network (NIPNET) is a network that fosters interprofessional collaboration in education, practice and research. It is primarily for Nordic educators, practitioners and researchers in the fields of health. NIPNET has the following aims: to explore theories and evidence for interprofessional education and collaboration; to develop approaches and methods for interprofessional learning and practice; to evaluate interprofessional education and practice activities; and stimulate exchange of ideas and experiences between the Nordic countries. Website: http://www.nipnet.org/

Patient Safety Network

Patient Safety Network (PSNet) is an initiative supported by the US Agency for Healthcare Research and Quality. It is a national web-based resource featuring the latest news and resources on patient safety. The site offers weekly updates of patient safety and teamwork literature, news, tools and meetings, and a set of links to research and other information on patient safety and team training and teamwork. Website: http://www.psnet.ahrq.gov/

Other useful teamwork links

Below is a short list of other useful website links which provide additional perspectives and ideas about teamwork.

Academic Health Council

The Academic Health Council (AHC) actively promotes the value and benefits of research and facilitation while promoting interprofessional care in the health services. It assists health and social care professions to learn, plan and work in a more interprofessional manner. Website: http://www.ahc-cas.ca/resources-e.php

Enhancing Interdisciplinary Collaboration in Primary Health Care

Funded by the Government of Canada through its Primary Health Care Transition Fund, the Enhancing Interdisciplinary Collaboration in Primary Health Care (EICP) initiative developed a website which offers a range of reports and resources on teamwork in primary health care. Website: http://www.eicp.ca/en/resources/articles.asp

Geriatric Interdisciplinary Team Training Program

Geriatric Interdisciplinary Team Training (GITT) Program Kit provides a step-by-step approach, focusing on lessons learned from the geriatric team experts. This kit can be used in shared work focused on improving geriatric interdisciplinary team training opportunities. The manual provides an overview of the GITT Program on how to develop, implement and evaluate GITT initiatives. Website: http://www.americangeriatrics.org/education/gitt/gitt.shtml

Journal of Interprofessional Care

The *Journal of Interprofessional Care* is the main journal for the worldwide dissemination of policy, evidence and theoretical perspectives informing collaboration in education and practice between medicine, nursing, veterinary science, allied health, public health, social care and related professions. Website: http://informahealthcare.com/jic

London Deanery

The London Deanery is an NHS-funded organisation working to improve the quality of patient care by ensuring the supply of doctors and dentists. Their website offers a range of open access modules. One module focuses on interprofessional learning in the clinical context, which considers the policies and contexts of interprofessional practice as well as how one can design and implement interprofessional learning activities aimed at promoting interprofessional teamwork. Website: http://www.faculty.londondeanery.ac.uk/e-learning/interprofessional-education

Regional Geriatric Program

The Regional Geriatric Program aims to support health care providers in the delivery of interdisciplinary and interprofessional, senior-friendly and evidence-based care which optimises the function and independence of seniors and supports ageing. The website offers a range of teaching and learning resources aimed at developing teamwork and interprofessional practice. Website: http://rgp.toronto.on.ca/

Index

Abstracted empiricism, 78
Academic Health Council, 187
Accreditation, 99, 102
Accreditation Council for Graduate Medical Education, 31
Action research, 97, 175
Activity theory, 84–5
American Interprofessional Health Collaborative (AIHC), 33, 185
American Physical Therapy Association, 31
Appreciative inquiry, xiv, 104
Asynchronous communication, xiv, 34, 63, 68
Audit Commission, 11
Australasian Interprofessional Practice and Education Network (AIPPEN), 33, 185

Benchmark statements. *See* Interprofessional education

Canadian Health Services Research Foundation, 2
Canadian Interprofessional Health Collaborative (CIHC), 33, 185
Care mapping, 68
Case management, xiv, 46, 97
Centre for the Advancement of Interprofessional Education (CAIPE), 33, 186
Chronic illness, 27–8
Collaboration, xiv. *See also* Interprofessional typology
Collaborative patient-centred care/practice, xiv, 26–7
Community mental health teams, 64, 73
Competency frameworks. *See* Interprofessional education
Complexity of clinical work, 69
Computer conferencing, xiv, 68
Consumerism, 29
Continuous quality improvement (CQI), xiv, 54, 102. *See also* Quality improvement initiatives
Crew resource management (CRM), xiv, 52–3, 96
Cultural issues, 72–4

Danish Medical Association, 31
Demographic shifts, 27–8
Department of Health (UK), 31
Department of Health and Human Services (US), 30
Descriptive studies, 112–13
Direct teamwork intervention, xiv, 93, 96, 100, 102
Discourse theory, 79, 88–9. *See also* Power
Diversity in teams, 74
Division of labour, 60

Economics
    Costs and effect, 75
    Economic rewards, 76
    Rising costs of health care, 29–30
Education. *See* Interprofessional education
Emotional labour, 63
Epistemology, xv, 79, 119
Ethnography, xv, 174
European Interprofessional Education Network, 186
Evaluation, xv
    Considerations, 105–7
    Critical appraisal tools, 180–81
    Critical approach to evaluation, 106
    Designing teamwork evaluations, 172–9
    Dissemination, 176
    Ethics, 177–8
    Evaluative tools, 182–4
    Formative, xv, 108–9
    Future directions, 142–3
    Mixed methods, xvi, 118–20, 142, 175
    Models, 172–3
    Nature of, 107–8
    Need for, 107
    Participation in, 117–8
    Planning checklist, 178–9
    Practicalities, 176–7
    Purpose of, 108–9
    Qualitative approaches, 115–18, 174–5
    Quantitative approaches, 112–14, 173–4
    Summative, xvii, 109
    Synthesizing evaluation studies, 121–36
    Targets, 110
    Type of evidence, 110–12
    Use of theory, 117
Expert patient programmes, xv, 29

Family health teams, 14–15
Formative evaluation. *See* Evaluation
Framework for interprofessional teamwork, 4, 8, 57–8, 79, 102
    Contextual factors, 4, 57–8, 72–6, 141
    Organisational factors, 4, 57–8, 70–72, 141
    Processual factors, 4, 57–8, 66–70, 141
    Relational factors, 4, 57–65, 141

Gender, 50, 74–5
General medicine teams, 85, 101, 126–32
Geriatric Interdisciplinary Team Training Program (GITT), 187

Grand theory, 78–9, 90
Groupthink, 64

Hawthorne effect. *See* Reactivity
Health Canada, 14, 27, 31
Hegemony, 59. *See also* Power
Hierarchy, 60–61
HIV teams, 16

Iatrogenic disease, 25
Impression management theory, 82–4
Indirect teamwork interventions, xv, 93, 96, 98, 102
Information technology, 33–4, 68
Institute for Healthcare Improvement (IHI), 18, 33, 54, 186
Institute of Medicine, 25, 30
Institutional influence theory, 79, 85–6
Integrated care pathways, xv, 96–7
Interactionism, xv, 79, 82–4
Interprofessional collaboration. *See* Interprofessional typology
Interprofessional coordination. *See* Interprofessional typology
Interprofessional education, xvi, 35–6, 82, 93–4
    Benchmark statements, xiv, 36
    Competency frameworks, 36
    Simulation, 94
    Teambuilding, 65, 93
    Team retreats, 94
Interprofessional Education for Collaborative Patient-Centred Practice (IECPCP), 14, 27
Interprofessional networks. *See* Interprofessional typology
Interprofessional teamwork, xvi
    Arguments for, 1–2
    Champions, 33, 134
    Conceptual issues, 3–4
    Contingency approach, 4, 7, 43–8, 138, 142
    Descriptions, 39–41
    Emergence, 12–18
    Funding for, 31–2
    Historical accounts, 15–17
    Key dimensions, 10–11
    Online resources, 185–8
    Professional experiences, 19–22
    Support for, 11–12
    Team performance factors, 48–51
    Team tasks, 40–2
    Underlying assumptions, 5–6
Interprofessional teamwork interventions, xvi
    Classification, 91–2
    Contextual interventions, 100, 102
    Design issues, 136, 141
    Developing and piloting, 115
    Implementation factors, 133–4
    Intervention activities, 168–71
    Intervention planning tools, 165–8
    Limitations, 103–4
    Multifaceted interventions, xvi, 100–102
    Organisational interventions, 98–100, 102
    Processual interventions, 96–8, 102
    Relational interventions, 93–6, 102

Use of theory, 103
Interprofessional typology, 44, 141–2
    Adaptive teamwork, 47, 138, 142
    Collaboration, xiv, 45–6, 124
    Comparing typologies, 48
    Coordination, 45–6
    Networking, 46–7
    Teamwork, 45, 124
Intervention studies, 113
Intraprofessional, xvi, 126

Joint Commission for Accreditation of Healthcare, 54
Journal of Interprofessional Care, 187

Kaiser Permanente, 18
Knotworking, 67, 85

Lay participation, 29, 35
Leadership. *See* Team roles
Litigation, fear of, 72
London Deanery, 188
Long-term care teams, 59, 81
Loss and change theory, 80–81

Magical thinking, 103–4
Magnet Hospital Initiative, 18, 99
Maternity care teams, 17
Media coverage, 28–9
Medical Home Model, 18
Medical Research Council, 165–6
Meta-ethnography, xvi, 125
    Key findings, interprofessional interaction, 125–32
Micro theory, 78–9
Mid-range theory, 78–9
Mind mapping, 171
Mixed methods. *See* Evaluation

National Health Service (NHS), 15–16
National Health Service Management Executive, 12
National Institute of Health Research (NIHR), 32
Negotiated order theory, 82–3
Nordic Interprofessional Network (NIPNET), 186
NorthStar, 167
Nurse practitioners. *See* Professional roles
Nursing and Midwifery Council, 26, 31

Operating room teams, 26, 95, 115
Organisational support for teams, 71

Palliative care teams, 61
Paradigms, xvi, 118–19
Patient-centred care, xvi, 25–6
    Medical homes, 18
Patient participation. *See also* Lay participation
    In evaluation studies, 117
Patient Safety Network (PSNet), 186
Patient safety
    Conflict and error, 25
    Patient safety agencies, 25
    Perceptions of error, 25–6
Patriarchy, xvi, 74–5
Physician assistants. See Professional roles

Political will, 75
Positivism, xvii, 118
Power
  Patient-professionals, 27, 29
  Professional, 59–60, 88–9
  Professions-management, 71
  Resistance, 60
Primary care teams, 34, 66, 70, 89, 98
Professional associations, 31, 71
Professional identity, 61
Professional roles
  Evolution, 35
  Nurse practitioners, 30, 70, 98
  Physician assistants, 30, 35, 70
  Role/task shifting, 69–70, 98, 102
  Specialisation, 35
  Working regulations, 35
Professional socialisation, 61, 82
Professionalisation theory, xvii, 86–8
Public inquiries, 28–9

Quality of care issues, 24–5
Quality improvement initiatives, xvii, 54–5, 99, 102
Qualitative methods. See Evaluation
Quantitative methods. See Evaluation

Randomised trials, xvii, 113, 173
Reactivity, 176
Realistic conflict theory, 81–2
Reflexivity, xvii, 5–6, 65, 139, 170
Registered Nurses Association of Ontario, 34
Reorganising the delivery of care, 99–100
Resistance. See Power
Reviews, xvii
  Scoping review, xvii, 91–2
  Systematic review, xvii, 30
Role shifting. See Professional roles
Routines and rituals, 67
Royal College of Nursing, 31
Royal College of Physicians and Surgeons of Canada, 36
Rural care, 30
  Rural mental health teams, 13

SBAR (Situation-Background-Assessment-Reccomendation), 95, 169–70
Social defence theory, 80
Social identity theory, 81–2
Socialisation. See Professional socialisation
Sports teams, 55–6, 87
Stereotypes, 61, 82
Stroke teams, 32
Summative evaluation. See Evaluation
SUPPORT tools, 166–7
Surveillance theory, 79, 88–9
Synchronous communication, xvii, 33–4, 63, 68

Task shifting. See Professional roles
Team checklists, 95

Team composition, 61–2
Team processes
  Communication, 63
  Conflict, 64
  Humour, 64
  Individual willingness, 65
  Teambuilding. See Interprofessional education
  Team emotions, 63
  Team stability, 65
  Trust and respect, 63–4
Team reflexivity. See Reflexivity
Team roles, 62
Teamwork activities/experiences
  Australia, 12–13, 19, 21
  Brazil, 13–14
  Canada, 13–15, 19, 21, 27, 36–7, 123–4, 126, 139–40
  Norway, 19, 21
  South Africa, 14–16, 20–2, 121–2, 124, 126
  United Kingdom, 15–17, 20, 22, 32, 37, 122–4, 126, 140
  United States, 16–18, 20, 22, 34, 37, 140
Teamwork in non-health care settings, 51–6
  Aircraft crews, 52–3
  Applications to health and social care, 53–6
  Quality improvement teams, 54
  Sports teams, 55
Teamwork leader perspectives, 36–8, 139–40
Temporal and spatial factors, 66–7
Terminological issues, 9, 91
Theories
  Implications, 88–90
  Limitations, 90
  Organisational theories, 79, 85–6
  Psychodynamic theories, 79–81
  Social psychological theories, 79, 81–2
  Sociological theories, 79, 82–4, 86–8
  Systems theories, 79, 84–5
  Theory building, 117
  Types of theory, 77–9
  Use of theories, 81–2, 84–5, 87, 89, 117
Total quality management, xvii, 54, 102. See also Quality improvement initiatives
Triangulation, xviii, 118

Unions, 71–2
Uniprofessional. See Intraprofessional
Unpredictability in teams, 68–9
Urgency of clinical work, 69

Validity, 113–14
Veterans Administration (VA), 17–18
Videoconferencing, xviii, 33–4

Wikipedia, xviii, 29
W.K. Kellogg Foundation, 17, 100
Work-group mentality theory, 80
World Health Organization, 25

CPSIA information can be obtained at www.ICGtesting.com
Printed in the USA
BVOW061344161212

308175BV00005B/25/P